Diary of a Prostate Wimp

the aftermath of having a prostate biopsy

Mike Crowl

Frank Joseph Publishing—Dunedin—New Zealand

Frank Joseph Publishing
127 Glenpark Avenue
Maryhill
Dunedin 9011 New Zealand
mcrowl@gmail.com

Paperback edition 2018 KDP ISBN 978-1-718-03265-1
First published by Frank Joseph Publishing in 2014 in e-book format

Cover and production design: Ben Crowl

to Charlie
who thought what I had to say was useful

and Dave
whose experiences were worse than mine

Auckland Urologist's Personalized Number Plate: NOPCME

I do not believe that sheer suffering teaches. If suffering alone taught, all the world would be wise, since everyone suffers. To suffering must be added mourning, understanding, patience, love, openness, and the willingness to remain vulnerable.

—Anne Morrow Lindbergh

CONTENTS

Chapter one

Like it or not, you need to read this to make sense of what comes later

Back in late 2008, I went to the doctor for a routine PSA checkup. PSAs offer a rough picture of the state of your prostate, as to whether it's behaving or not. The higher the number on your PSA, the more likely it is that your prostate is going to cause you some trouble. More about PSAs later.

Not long after this checkup, I fronted up for an appointment at our local hospital's Urology Department. As a result of a digital examination (more about those later, too) the urologist decided I should have a biopsy, in case I had prostate cancer. This book is the story of what happened after that, and of my emotional ups and downs. Being a bit of a wimp, I had plenty of ups and downs, but such feelings aren't actually uncommon to men faced with anything happening to their prostates, since the prostate resides in such a strategic area of a man's body.

In 2008, I was writing a blog called WorkReport.net. Since the biopsy and prostate stuff affected my work, I decided to include the occasional post about the situation. The prostate posts became more and more frequent and detailed, and eventually attracted the attention of an Australian by the name of Charlie, who told me, "*I am a lot better informed regarding the problem than I would have been had I not found your blog by accident.*" I replied to him, and we kept up a correspondence about his situation and mine, and we still keep in touch today. His encouragement gave me the idea of turning the blog posts into a book.

Being the sort of person who tends to write almost as much as I breathe, I've also been keeping a journal—or diary—for many years, and naturally the prostate process made its way into that as well. I've also been writing what I call "God Notes" most mornings since the 1970s. These are a kind of ongoing discussion I have with God about my life and what I'm doing with it.

When putting this book together I decided to combine the blog posts, the journal and the God Notes, since they each add a different element to the overall picture. So there are three slightly different voices in this book talking about the same situation. The blog posts are the most upbeat and breezy, while the journal notes, like any diary, vary from day to day.

A lot of what I wrote in the God Notes during the time I was having prostate issues was where the Wimp came into his own. However, the Psalmists in Scripture spent a good deal of time whining about their situations too, so I felt justified in my grumbling. You can ignore these notes if you want. If you've had anything go wrong with your prostate, you may think that compared to what's happened—or what may be happening—to you, I sound like a big baby. You're possibly right.

I learned about prostates and biopsies and PSAs and much more as I went along. So what I talk about early in the book is often clarified later. Google was very helpful when I discovered that I didn't know enough, and as I've put this book together, I've learned still more. There may be comments here that aren't technically or medically completely accurate, for which I apologize in advance. This isn't meant to be a medical book; it's a sharing of experience.

In the 7 April entry I write: *I think men facing anything to do with their prostate should talk to as many men as possible about what's likely to happen, and what can happen. You find, once you start opening your mouth to other guys, that there's a lot more information out there than you thought.*

I discovered there were plenty of men out there willing to share their information. I didn't have to look far: cousins, in-laws, friends. Many of them had experienced some issue with their prostates, and the things that can happen when medicos start fiddling around with it. One person in particular, Dave, had written a good deal on his own blog about his prostate experiences, and he's given me permission to include extracts from that blog in this book. This adds a fourth voice to the mix. Dave is no wimp, but he's also had some very low moments.

Most importantly you need to remember that what follows is *my* experience, and isn't by any means the experience of every man confronted with prostate issues. Many men get through prostate biopsies and operations without much difficulty, others follow a path similar to mine, and some, regrettably, have worse experiences. Whatever the situation, it's essential that you check your PSA with your doctor regularly, especially as you reach middle-age. At present, the PSA blood test is the best indicator we have that anything is amiss with the prostate, and biopsies are currently the best means of finding out whether you have prostate cancer or not. It's better to find out earlier than later when it comes to prostate cancer.

What I don't want this book to do is put any man off getting PSA tests or biopsies. What I hope it will do is help you to ask questions about your situation, and encourage you to talk to other men who've gone through a prostate biopsy and operation. They've been there—many doctors haven't—and they're worth listening to.

A couple of other notes: the abbreviation GP is used several times in this book. In New Zealand, and a number of other countries, it stands for General Practitioner, a family doctor who is part of a private practice. In some other countries, including the USA, General Practitioner may have a slightly different meaning.

I also mention District Nurses. These are trained nurses who visit patients in their own homes, and liaise with the hospital system.

I've sometimes included a few comments from people who wrote in response to particular blog posts. These are generally comments that were important—or amusing— at the time. Now on with the story.

Chapter two

Pretending a health issue doesn't exist won't make it go away

Work Report
28 October 2008
Working on the Prostate

Today was memorable. For the second time in two or three years I had an appointment at the hospital to have a prostate check.

Doctors keep an eye on the state of prostates by using blood tests that give them a PSA reading. PSA means Prostate-Specific Antigen, if that's any help to you. Apparently it's something that the prostate exudes into the bloodstream as a matter of course. The blood test can tell whether its level is normal or not.

As guys get older, the PSA number goes up. For my age, sixty-three, it should only be around four or five. Mine is ten, however, and has been climbing slowly for a few years. At my previous prostate examination, the hospital doctor decided not to do a biopsy, for which I was grateful. He performed a digital examination. This itself is invasive enough, though short. Basically the doctor sticks a finger up your rear end and fiddles around, finds the prostate, and roughly determines its size.

Anyway, today's digital examination was survivable, but the doctor said that because of the high number on my tests, I should now have a biopsy. He didn't really give me a lot of choice about the matter, and mentioned the word "cancer" a few times, just to make sure he was going to get his way.

So I'm due for a biopsy sometime in the next few months.

I rang my GP when I got back to work, and asked if the number my blood tests were producing was necessarily indicative of cancer. She said, "No, it can also indicate a benign prostatic hyperplasia" (that tongue-twister is usually reduced to BPH. You could remember it by the phrase: Better Pee Hurriedly.)

In layman's terms BPH is essentially an increase in the size of the prostate. It's a fairly normal process that happens to the majority of men as they grow older. When the prostate isn't enlarged, it sits comfortably around the urethra (the tube from the bladder to the penis that urine flows through), and the two do their work without annoying each other. But as nodules gradually form (from middle-age onwards) and enlarge the prostate, the urethra gets squashed, like a tube of toothpaste being squeezed with someone's fist. The result is that the urine from the bladder can't flow so easily. Peeing becomes a stop-start process, there's a need to pee more often, and sometimes an increase in infections. However, this enlargement of the prostate isn't necessarily an indication of prostate cancer; it's a process of age, and mainly more annoying than anything.

I don't have much in the way of urine flow problems. In fact this area seems to be currently better than it used to be, possibly as a result of a tablet (Hytrin) I've been taking for the past few years, which is aimed at keeping things flowing.

It doesn't really pay to start looking up what happens when a biopsy is performed, but I looked up Wikipedia anyway, and discovered that in a prostate biopsy small samples are taken from the prostate gland so they can be tested for cancer.

It's something that's done in the Outpatients' Department of your hospital, and it requires a local anesthetic. Often there's bleeding in the urine for a few days; occasionally bleeding in the feces and some blood in ejaculations. The latter may last for a few weeks, though I'm not sure how many men would notice. Antibiotics are given to eliminate infection.

The biopsy is normally performed through the anus, sometimes up through the urethra (yup, that's up through the penis), and more rarely through the perineum, the area between the testicles (or scrotum) and the anus. I'm not sure why this latter approach would be taken since it sounds quite dangerous, but perhaps other complications would make it the only option.

In the common transrectal approach (via the anus, that is), an ultrasound probe is inserted to guide the urologist in his or her task. The prostate is given an anesthetic, and finally a thin spring-loaded prostate tissue collection needle is inserted through the rectum and into the prostate about a dozen times. It takes six samples from each side of the prostate.

The Wikipedia writer talked about the anesthetic being "similar to the local anesthetic administered for a dental procedure." That's supposed to be encouraging? I avoid anesthetics at the dentist's, if I can help it. They cause the pain to be prolonged, I find.

Fifty-five percent of men, according to the writer, report "considerable discomfort" during the biopsy. What do the other forty-five percent report? We're not told; perhaps it's because they pass out in the middle of it all! A man's comfort isn't helped by the sharp clicking that goes on during the procedure. The digital examination I had today itself caused considerable discomfort, the only consolation being that it was quick.

Anyway, enough of all this. Just had to jot it down in order to get some of the tension it was causing out of my head!

Maybe I should wear a t-shirt: "I survived yet another rectal examination."

Since I wrote this I've discovered that the practice of transrectal biopsy is becoming increasingly questioned in the medical profession because of the considerable risk of infection from the rectum. In spite of antibiotics, it's possible for bacteria from the rectum to infect the prostate, urethra and bladder areas, and this has been known to sometimes cause massive complications. In a number of cases, men have died through sepsis—the transmittal of bacteria to the bloodstream.

In spite of my saying in my original post that a biopsy through the perineum would be a dangerous approach, it's now being seen as a healthier option, because there should be no risk of bacteria from the anus. Presumably considerable caution has to be taken not to interfere with other vital parts of the male anatomy. The procedure is done under heavier sedation, with several people in the operating theatre—and of course it costs more.

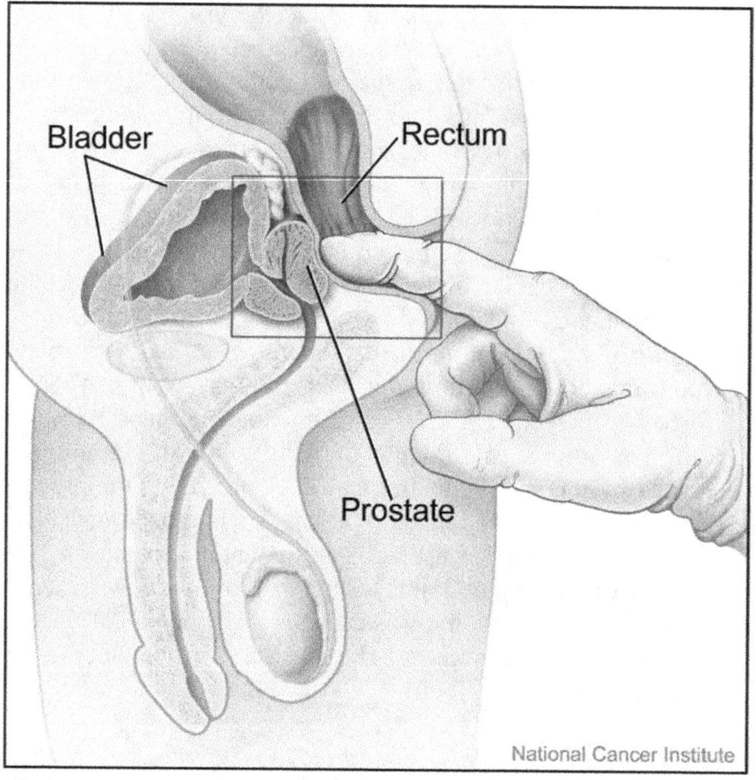

This picture shows the digital rectal check: it looks quite easy here. Note too that there's a lining between the rectum and the prostate which the needle has to penetrate in a biopsy.

God Notes
29 October 2008

[In the God Notes I often address God as "Dad." This might seem a bit familiar, but Jesus called God *Abba*, an Aramaic word for "Father," so I'm just following in his footsteps.]

Well, Dad, you know how I've dropped from having a sense of ease right down into tensions and concerns, all because of something that hasn't even happened yet, something that may not in fact be much of a problem. Yet even my GP's reassurances yesterday may not be quite as reassuring as they seemed. The BPH side of things may still mean there's something growing on the prostate, and I guess *that* means the prostate may have to be removed as well. Dad, I just don't know what I'm thinking. Having the guy yesterday going on about the possibility of cancer was pretty undermining of my confidence, even though it's not conclusive, and presumably the biopsy will give us something more definite. But basically, Dad, I'm just scared underneath. I seem to have lost trust and security in you, all in a moment—I feel as though I'm trying to manage on my own, and of course I'm *not* managing.

All the Psalms in the section I'm currently reading talk about *men* doing nasty things to the psalmist, not about your own flesh doing nasty things to *itself*.

Be gracious to me, O God my Father
For my soul takes refuge in you.
I will hide in the shadow of your wings
Until destruction passes by. [Psalm 57:1—my paraphrase]

Dad, I know it's not our lot to live forever: I look out on the garden, or think of Celia [my wife] saying, "I've never really known you to be ill," or think of our grandchildren growing up and me not being here, and I feel a sense of great loss. I'm sure I'm hardly alone in this, but it's something I'm finding hard to face all the same.

I see all sorts of other people suffering, and my first thought is *thank goodness that's not me,* and I lack sympathy for what they're going through. Do I really lack empathy to such a degree? Perhaps I do.

This isn't confession so much as trying to get a sense of realism about myself, and my general selfishness. If it concerns *me*, it's of great concern; if it concerns others, I'm very casual about it. Or so it often seems. Dad, you know the truth of it all.

Anyway, here I am, struggling a good deal to come to terms with what might be a period of pain and/or the beginning of the end of things as I know them.

Dad, we all die—none of us, somehow, thinks it's real. It happens to others, not us. It seems pointless, wasteful, useless. Dad, help me to get some sense on it all.

I've since learned that both a cousin and a friend of mine have each had this invasive biopsy twice. The friend seemed rather blasé about it; the cousin had some bleeding from his penis the second time which "freaked him out a little."

For me it was the cancer factor I was most concerned about, though that turned out to be the least of my problems. However I still remember walking back from the hospital in a daze as though I'd been told I did have cancer. All I'd had was a bit of a fright. Such is the way the mind plays tricks.

Work Report
29 October 2008
Pity Me Prostate

Well, I did the "pity me" stuff (pity me prostate!) for most of last night and some of this morning, and then somehow perked up again and carried on with life.

Celia reckons I'm more of an optimist than I give myself credit for, especially in some areas of life. As we agreed this morning, nothing has actually changed since yesterday. I haven't had any nasty biopsies as yet, and haven't had any actual bad news (just threats of it - and sticks and stones may break my bones, and nasty needles may poke my prostate, but threats will never hurt me).

I must say I'd sooner have several more PSAs (these only require a blood sample) than any further fiddling around with the rear end, but if it must be, it must be. I've had a very healthy life, all up. Never been in hospital for more than a couple of nights (and that was a false alarm), and never broken any bones or chopped off any important parts.

Part of my healing process today was that I had lunch with an old friend who told me he's going to audition as an extra for *Kingdom Come*, a new film about Jesus that's being shot up in Central Otago early next year. They're looking for males and females from eight to eighty, the adult men preferably with beards. I have a beard. I've always had an ambition to be involved in a movie, so I'm going to go along with him and see what happens. Might have to take a bit of time off work if I get in (probably as unpaid leave), but we'll sort that out when it comes.

Central Otago is a large area inland from where I live in the coastal city of Dunedin. Very hot in the summer, often very frosty in the winter. Queenstown is its major town, a heavily-populated place, and a Mecca for tourists and the self-proclaimed "undisputed adventure capital of the world."

God Notes
30 October 2008

Well, Dad, feeling a lot less focused on the prostate issue today—and most of yesterday. Need to get on with life as it *is*, and deal with the prostate business when it has its day.

God Notes
1 November 2008

Thank you, Dad, that I felt better most of yesterday as far as my back was concerned. It's a bit of a puzzle, this whole thing of feeling as though I've strained my neck and upper back somehow. I can only conclude it's from sitting badly somewhere recently. Dad, it would be good if it would clear up of its own accord.

Work Report
1 November 2008
Continuing to talk about health: *I attend a casting call*

By Wednesday, I'd kind of come to grips with the idea that I was going to have to have a biopsy on my prostate at some time in the near future, so I was feeling mostly normal again. On Thursday, however, I woke up with a pain in my side, sort of around the upper ribs, and my upper back seemed tight, as though it was being compressed slightly. And then my neck got in on the act and complained of being stiff and irritated.

I half-jokingly said at work that it was probably "third-day stress," a reaction to the news I'd received on Tuesday. On Friday morning it was still there and then cleared up fairly quickly. On Friday evening the neck thing returned, and still hasn't really gone away entirely.

It may well be stress. Who knows. It might be a bit of a bug. Let's hope it clears up anyway; it's annoying!

Meanwhile, the casting call for *Kingdom Come* was looming up. And last night I dreamt about it at length, about all the things they might ask me to do to prove I should be in the movie.

The reality was that it was only a casting call, with no auditioning required whatsoever. Can't imagine why I dreamt there should be.

Anyway, I went along this morning with my friend, and apart from having to stand in the queue for a while, the thing was a breeze. Admittedly they were looking for people who could pass for Arabs or Jews or Middle Easterners, and while there were a few of those around, the crowd was pretty varied. Plenty of Europeans, for starters.

Anyway, we had to take off our shoes before we got in the main door--not because of any cultural issues, but because they wanted us to draw around one of our feet to give them an idea of foot size. This was done on the back of the application form.

Once the form was filled in, there was nothing else to do except pose for a photo while holding a board with your name scribbled on it. Three or four shots were taken and then we were out of there. One of the women in charge said to me, "Keep growing that beard." I could assume all sorts of things from that, but I'll wait for some confirmation before I start getting excited.

So there we go: my first ever casting call. Thrilling.

The casting call for Kingdom Come *never came to anything. In fact, even though a village set was built near Lake Benmore (in Central Otago), it was never used, and the film appears to have been abandoned.*

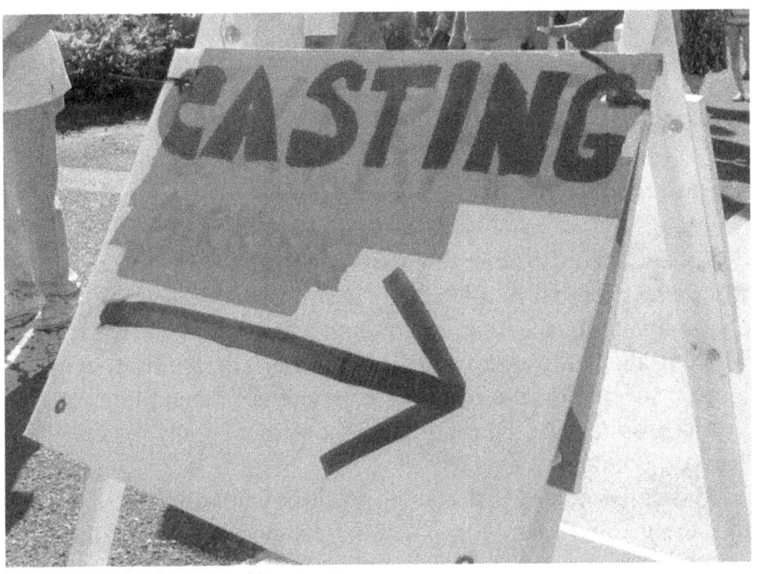

God Notes
4 November 2008

Going to see my GP today and instead of feeling reassured I'm feeling all shaky again, as though something drastic was in the offing. Help me to trust you in all this, Dad. I can't seem to get you in focus and certainly am not at rest in you. Feel almost as bad, since I got up, as I did when I was in my worst day at the shop. Which is silly. Understandable, but silly nevertheless. Give me your peace, Dad. If I'm like this now, I'll be a nervous wreck when the biopsy comes round.

I'd managed a Christian bookshop for seventeen years, and the entire time it struggled financially—not because of incompetence on my part, but because customers no longer bought the breadth of materials they once had, and because Internet bookselling was on the rise, and because of changes in the bookselling culture in general. Some nights I'd wake with panic attacks, and more than once I was on anti-depressants. I finally resigned in 2006. The shop's Board took over, appointed another manager, who struggled as much as I did, and eventually the shop closed in 2008.

Work Report
4 November 2008
Visit to the Doctor: *quailing at the thought*

I mentioned the other day that I'd felt I'd been suffering a bit from stress, probably related to the prostate business. I made an appointment to see my doctor and went today. I wasn't too worried about the stress stuff; the more I thought about it the more it seemed to be a reaction to concerns I'd had after my visit to the hospital last Tuesday, and the urologist saying the word 'cancer' a number of times.

Basically today I just wanted to sit down with the doctor and talk the whole thing over, get some perspective on it. I did that: asked questions, got answers—when she could give them—and was taken seriously and listened to, which is always a plus. Don't know that I learned anything new. Had a number of things confirmed, and listened again to some of the more unpleasant factors that might be involved at some point.

If the prostate does prove to have any cancerous cells (not in itself a life-threatening matter) and they decide to remove it, they somehow *take it out through the penis.* Now this is enough to make any male quail. I'd think even the doctors doing it must quail. My GP assured me this is done under general anesthetic, but I'm not sure that helps.

Anyway, we're going to have to face that if and when it comes. In the meantime, the biopsy, according to my doctor, is still somewhat a matter of choice. I had another PSA blood test done today, and if that shows stability since the last test, then it's possible we'll do a "wait and see" approach. If it's gone up further from last time, then it will pretty much confirm that there's something needing attention, and a biopsy will be the next step. It may also depend on the urologist's report from the hospital, which hasn't reached my GP yet.

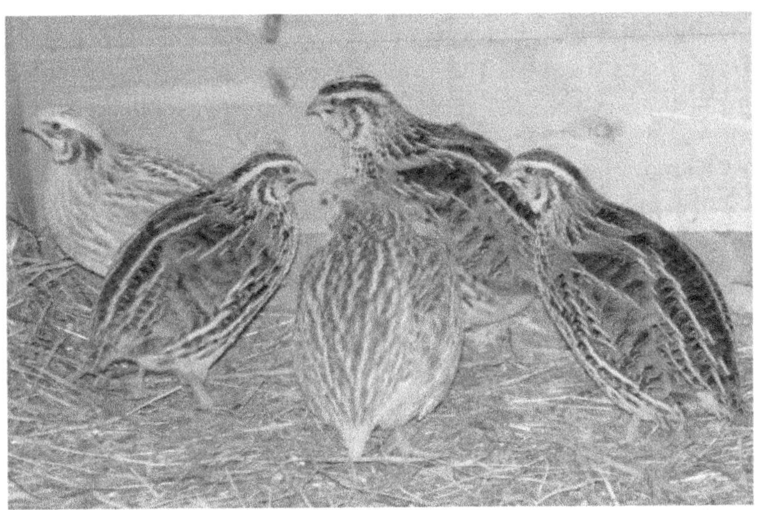

Quail showing no obvious signs of quailing

God Notes
5 November 2008

Dad, thank you for the conversation with my GP yesterday. It was worth having even though it probably told me nothing new. Except that there were still some options rather than just a *fait accompli*.

But what then was the groin pain that seemed to come out of nowhere? It's one strange pain after another at the moment. Perhaps it's all reaction stuff. Hopefully I'll get some peace about it all, in the same way I've been praying for peace for others.

"Who do you know who really knows you, knows your heart? And even if they did, is there anything they would discover in you that you could take credit for? Isn't everything you have, and everything you are, sheer gifts from God?" [1 Corinthians 4:7, The Message]

Work Report
8 November 2008
Trying not to harp on: *always look on the bright side*

Without wishing to harp on about the prostate business I've been discussing over the last couple of weeks, I'm going to mention it again. This time, hopefully, from a more positive viewpoint.

Nothing has so far changed on the prostate side, except that the latest blood test, done last Wednesday, showed that the PSA level had risen yet again, to eleven point something.

Anyway, sometime this week I came to the conclusion that focusing on the future from a negative point of view wasn't the way to go. Obvious, really, but sometimes it takes a bit to get to such a point.

I need to think about whether the coming year is going to be one of holding back - primarily because of the prostate thingee— or one of achieving some things. So I'd still like to float some possibilities for next year. The Good Lord can deal with them or not as he sees fit.

Here they are:

- maybe being an extra in the movie;
- maybe doing a paper on Research for University through distance learning;
- maybe doing the week-long block course on Congregations in New Zealand, at University;
- maybe putting on another concert of my more-recently-composed music;
- maybe acting in the next Narnia play (*The Silver Chair*), if there's something suitable;
- maybe acting in a friend's production of *A Christmas Carol*, if it gets off the ground;
- and no doubt other things…

All these are better things to focus on than bemoaning my fate. Maybe I will have a biopsy soon and the results will not be positive. Maybe I will have to have my prostate removed. I say a loud **YUCK** to that. But rather than making that the focus of life in 2009, let me focus on the positive things, and the prostate will just have to fit in around them.

God Notes
9 November 2008

Well, Dad, it's been a hectic few days, with some groin pain added to everything else, but now even that seems to be being put in its place.

Dad, I wrote last night on the blog about aiming for the things I could do in 2009 rather than what I might not be able to do. I know the list isn't necessarily stuff that helps others, reaches out, preaches the kingdom—at least not obviously. But it's all stuff for which I have a passion, and you know that you've given me all this stuff as a gift to work with. It's this old and constant argument I have with myself about what's of value—in the end it's what's of value to *you*. Does what I do please you? Is it what you made me for? Please somehow make it clear if I'm totally off the rails.

But it still seems better to me to spend a time of trial planting trees than lying down in my sick bed.[*I think this is a reference to something Martin Luther is supposed to have said, which is variously quoted along the lines of "Even if I knew the world would end tomorrow, I would still plant an apple tree today."*]

God Notes
10 November 2008

Dad, after yesterday's long walk I wound up with this groin pain and testicle tenderness again. Can it just be related to hauling spade-loads of dirt around on the weekend? Why only on that side—or is it just because that's always been the side that's had problems? It's very peculiar—hopefully it's *not* connected to the prostate stuff.

Dad, I think part of my concern is I'm truly afraid of death, of dying. I don't seem either to have the confidence in you to get me through it, or the confidence that you'll be there to keep me eternally, or that I'm in any way "right" enough to be yours forever. I feel very lacking in value in this way these days, Dad. I feel as though my life hasn't got much to show for it—plenty of hay, little precious metal. [*This is a reference to 1 Corinthians 3:12-15*] And I don't seem to be improving in that way.

Dad, does anyone want to leave this world? I guess those suffering hugely here probably do, but I can hardly be said to be a great sufferer. Does anyone whose life is pretty reasonable or good, as in general mine is, want to go somewhere unknown, however great a place it might be painted—especially if we've got to die to get there? Here's the selfish Crowl coming out: put it all off as long as possible. Is that my motto? All this scare stuff with the prostate is bringing to the fore things I don't want to think about. But I should keep them in view, all the same. Not that I've ever totally ignored them. I just don't like the idea, I think, of them seriously affecting me, giving me a fright.

Dad, I'm not very clear here. Help me to get my mind in a settled place.

When I was in my early thirties I had some severe pains in my left testicle and the groin area above it. The specialist told me to get on and live with it; just not to jump off tables, or go horse-riding, neither of which I normally did.

The groin pain, whatever it is, continues to turn up irregularly even today. It's just one of those pains you live with, and it doesn't appear to cause any damage elsewhere.

Work Report
13 November, 2008
The Continuing Saga: *what's the toilet seat got to do with it?*

My latest blood test was up another point on the PSA, which isn't good. So when I went to see the GP again this week—on a matter not related to the prostate—she said it looks as though getting the biopsy done is the best thing. The wisest thing, in fact.

I'll live through it, no doubt. At the moment I've been distracted by an odd groin pain that's come and gone over the last ten days. It's been worst when I've gone for a long walk, of all things. Anyway, it seems to be subsiding, and the doctor says it ain't a hernia, or an infection (a urine test showed that apparently), and it doesn't appear to be anything else particularly serious. So we're just getting through it and looking forward to the next health quirk. I go from one to another these last few months.

I picked up a book in the library today by Brian Turner (a writer from the UK, not the New Zealand poet) called *Please Leave the Seat Up!: Confronting my Prostate Cancer with Humor.* I haven't really had a good look at it yet. I'm mostly interested to know how they did the prostate operation in the end, in his case. Doubt it'll be that humorous, but one can live in hope!

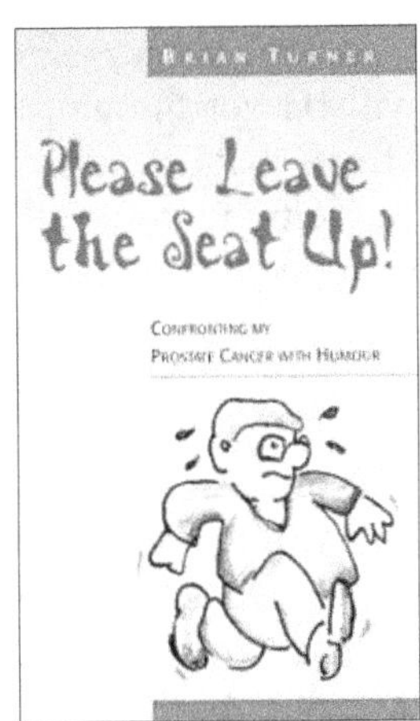

Since I never mentioned this book again, I suspect I never actually read very much of it—maybe it was too close to the bone at the time. Brian Turner died in 2007, four years after his prostate cancer operation.

God Notes
14 November 2008

However much I may want to put the prostate thing to the back of my mind it keeps coming forward again. So the verse in 1 Corinthians 13:7 (in *The Message* translation) which says, "Love trusts God always," is one I find difficult to grasp in the light not so much of the probable operation, but of the side effects, especially the possible loss of sexual function. It could be said that losing that would force me to stop worshipping it. That's assuming that I do "worship" it. Certainly it's been an ongoing battleground in my life, for much of my life.

Okay, loss of it would mean physical love would be something altogether different, which might be a good thing. But being who I am, it isn't easy for me to see how it can be. This is where trusting you, Dad, comes heavily into it. People all over the world lose a bodily function, sight, hearing, limbs, all manner of things, and have to live without them. And what Jesus says about it being better to lose some faculty rather than losing eternal life is relevant, for me, I suspect. [*This is a reference to Mark 9:43-48.*]

I think this aspect of it is my greatest fear—the pain side of it will be got through as most pain usually is. It's the long-term effects that I'm struggling with.

Help me to see all this, Dad, without bitterness or depression, or anger at you. I need to know that whatever happens I'm still in your hands; I'm still who you made me to be.

Work Report
15 November 2008
Hot and Productive Day

The groin pain I mentioned the other day is still niggling, though not seriously. It's a bit of a puzzle as to what's going on, but at present I'm just having to live with it. The worse thing about it is that it makes me feel just enough under the weather not to be able to get on with normal things...unless I really put my mind to it.

And there's been no news from the urology department; apparently speed in reporting back is not one of their strengths.

Anyway, it's been a scorcher of a day here, the sort of day that makes you remember what summer is all about, but so hot that you wouldn't really want to live with it day in and day out— at least we Dunedinites probably wouldn't. We like our weather a little less bright and burning.

Work Report
3 December 2008
Paellas and prostates

For those who might have been reading about my prostate issues in recent days, here's an update. Celia rang me today. She works in a health centre, and so has slightly more access to some of the hospital information than the man in the street, such as the man who's her husband. She'd contacted them to see if there was any news of an appointment, and the receptionist at the urology department said they'd had a cancellation, and they'd been trying to contact me—at my old phone number, the one for the bookstore, where I haven't been for two years!

So I go for a *biopsy tomorrow*. Think I must be in denial, as I'm not really too fazed about it. We'll see how I feel in the morning!

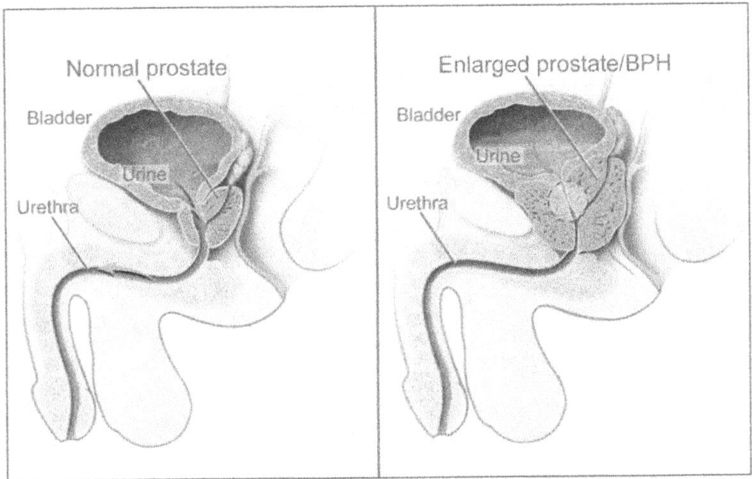

The normal prostate on the left, and an enlarged one on the right.
The latter shows how the urethra gets squeezed by the prostate.

I mentioned Dave in the Introduction to this book, as a kind of fourth voice who'll be appearing every now and then. While putting this book together, I happened to get in touch with him about something unrelated to prostates, and during the conversation discovered he was more than familiar with prostate problems. In his blog, on the 10 January 2012, he wrote:

Dave:

Today I go to hospital for a biopsy. The blurb from the day surgery unit at the hospital calls it a "procedure." Translated, that means they are going to do horrible things to me. It says there will be "mild discomfort." Translated, that means it's going to hurt like hell. They tell me I will not be able to drive home and I have to be with "a responsible adult" for 24 hours. I had a biopsy a few years ago and it was not a nice experience. I was talking to an older man the other day and it seems like I'll be having one every few years from now till when I die. That is, of course, if they don't discover prostate cancer in the process.

I've included Dave's comment here to show that it's not at all uncommon for men to feel concerned about having such procedures. The fact that the urinary system and the sexual apparatus are so intertwined adds to the concern. I know there are men who don't get uptight about such procedures. But those who do shouldn't feel they're any less of a man.

So, let's have a look at what happened to me next.

Chapter three

From confidence to confusion

Work Report
4 December 2008
The Great Biopsy: *waiting for more than one thing*

My prostate biopsy appointment was for 12.30 pm today. Being one of those people who can't help being early, I was there in plenty of time, and was out of my clothes and into the hospital open-backed gown (and a dressing gown, thank goodness) by the time 12.30 arrived. I should have been "done" and finished by 1 pm, but something went wrong. I think the head of the department, who was supposed to be involved in the biopsy, got caught up on an operation, and so all his afternoon patients got held up as well. Several of us were sitting in our open-backed hospital gowns and dressing gowns (and cuddly slippers) waiting, and waiting.

He and another urologist finally arrived about 1.45, or maybe later, after we'd all watched a dozen nurses, doctors, office workers and sundry other people walk back and forth carrying bits of paper and ticking things off on them, or making themselves cuppas or drinking water out of the water fountain. None of them actually told us what was happening. Once they were functioning with the doctors later on, they were very good; but a bit of communication during the waiting period wouldn't have gone amiss.

However, I must say that the nurse who was in charge of me most of the time was excellent, and friendly. But between initially sorting me out and the actual procedure, she had to go off to lunch. However, when she got back she stuck by me well and truly.

Now, if you're having a prostate biopsy, you're supposed to retain at least "a half bladderful" of urine. How you gauge a half bladderful is beyond me, but I'd dutifully not gone to the toilet for a while before I arrived. That would have been fine if my biopsy had been done on time, but having to hang on for another hour or more was fatal. Under normal circumstances if I don't go to the toilet when I really need to, the bladder muscles seize up, and it becomes very uncomfortable trying to get started.

For instance, a couple of years ago I was on a bus going to Christchurch. I should have asked the driver to let me have a minute to go to the toilet when we stopped in Ashburton, which is about an hour before Christchurch, but I didn't. And suffered for it. Usually on such an occasion things will eventually come right, but only after a very uncomfortable struggle. The same thing happened one night when we went to see *The Lion, the Witch and the Wardrobe* at the movies. It turned out to be longer than I expected, and by the time we got out I was desperate to go to the toilet, but could only manage a trickle. At that time, of course, I didn't realize the prostate was starting to squeeze the urethra.

Anyway, today I finally got into the operating theatre, where I was privileged to have one Ugandan nurse, one pregnant nurse, and another less conspicuous nurse (she was out of my sightline most of the time), plus Alistair, who did the biopsy. The Head of Department was also in the room, presumably to supervise, but he seemed preoccupied with paperwork. That was okay. I'd met him before when he did a rectal examination three years or so back, and didn't find him very user-friendly. Alistair was fine, and along with the nurses, he gave me a blow-by-blow account of what was happening. The most painful thing was having the ultrasound moving around inside; the actual chipping away of the bits of the prostate seemed far less uncomfortable.

By the time they'd done the procedure, however, I was desperate to go to the loo. And that was fine by the nurses, who wanted me to, in order to check my urine/blood levels. You may remember that a biopsy leaves you peeing a bit of blood in your urine for a few days.

However, it wasn't fine by my system, which literally and painfully seized up as though it was having a pregnancy contraction every time I tried to go. I dripped a few drops of blood, but that was all.

And what happens when you can't pee, however desperate you may be to do so? Well, if you're in the urology day surgery ward, they eventually use an in-out catheter (also called an intermittent catheter). And while the relief is enormous, putting the anesthetic *into* your penis is most unpleasant.

I note that on the Wikipedia entry on urinary catheterization, the writer says that for "some patients the insertion and removal of a catheter causes excruciating pain." Yup, he's right on the button there.

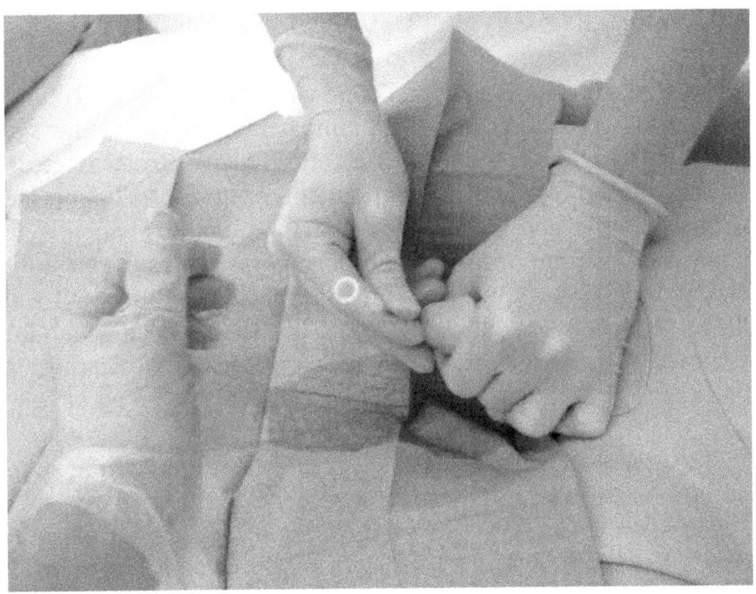

Insertion of a catheter—using a model, thankfully.

Having a wife who's worked with old people in rest homes, and in their own homes, I was familiar with the fact that if a man is going to have a catheter, it will be pushed up the opening in his penis. I'd said to Celia on more than one occasion over the years that I never wanted that to happen to me, that I couldn't imagine anything worse. Well, I no longer had to imagine.

However, the in-out catheter is a short moment of pain, and something of a shock to the system, but turns out to be well and truly worth the trouble.

Pain is a most odd thing. You anticipate it, but it's never anything like what you anticipate, because the imagination doesn't seem to be able to conjure up the actual feelings. Perhaps this is because it carefully puts pain memories away in the remote parts of the brain as soon as it can. It's always worse than you think, but if it's short-lived, it's bearable. I don't know much about long-term pain, which I imagine is another kettle of fish.

Anyway, I'm now past the biopsy pain, and the catheter pain. And the inability-to-pee pain. I live to fight another day.

God Notes
5 December 2008

Well, the biopsy is over and done with, thank you, Dad, and I can get on with life again for the time being. Thank you for my being able to get in because of a cancellation—that was great. Thank you too for my being able to cope better than I expected with the biopsy and the catheter in and out, both of which were unpleasant, but are now over and done with. I did struggle a bit at the time, especially with the unexpected waiting and the inability to pee, but thank you, we got there. Thank you for whoever discovered the catheter approach to clearing a blockage—it's unpleasant, but very effective!

I was told by Alistair at a much later date that in the past, when someone had this problem with not being able to pee—it's called water retention—they used to cut through the perineum to empty the bladder. You'll probably remember the perineum is the area between the testicles and the anus. I asked him how successful it was. "Not very," he said, "the patients often died."

And the man who invented the catheter that's used in most hospitals and surgeries around the world was Frederic Foley. The catheter is named after him.

God Notes
8 December 2008
Still a bit achy from last week, but surviving.

Work Report
9 December 2008
On the Prostate Front: *bad news and good news*

After the biopsy last Thursday, things came right pretty quickly. Friday was good: I felt like a box of birds. Saturday and Sunday were okay. Although things weren't completely up to the mark body-wise, I was still able to cope with them. Nothing serious.

On Sunday morning I got up out of bed and did twenty minutes on the treadmill at home, and felt fine. On Monday morning I did the same, had breakfast, and then suddenly had absolutely no energy whatsoever. Furthermore, my body, particularly my legs, felt as though I'd just run a marathon, rather than walking a couple of kilometers (just over a mile) on the treadmill. The treadmill doesn't usually wear me out that much.

I dragged myself off to work, but only lasted till lunchtime, when I was so weary that I could hardly keep awake. Came home and went straight to bed and fell into a deep sleep. Went to the doctor the next morning and she thought I might have a urinary tract infection, something that's not uncommon after a prostate biopsy. I'd had antibiotics for the effects of the biopsy but the course had already finished. She put me on another round of antibiotics and sent me home to bed. Ached and slept. And then about two in the afternoon found I was having trouble peeing again. By three I was wanting to go regularly—like every few minutes—but was finding it harder and harder. Shades of the post-biopsy problem.

Celia came and picked me up and took me back to the Health Clinic at about five. The doctor said there was nothing for it but to send me down to the Emergency Department to have another in-out catheter. *Oh, the joy.*

And of course, the Emergency Department isn't geared up to having someone arrive with a relatively minor ailment—like not being able to pee—and getting on and sorting it out straight away. Even though I probably didn't have to wait for more than an hour and a half, which was bad enough, I was still in considerable discomfort. My body wanted to pee, but it was impossible, and caused major seize-ups all round. I was sweating and tensed up.

Eventually I was sorted out, but this time the doctor recommended leaving the catheter in for a few days, in case the same problem occurred. *More joy*. Fortunately Celia knows all about dealing with catheters. On my own I would have been a mess in more ways than one. As it was I managed to empty the bag over my foot this morning.

So, after a night of sleeping with the day bag running into the night bag (this is used in case of an overflow), and this morning feeling quite uncomfortable every time I took a step – it looks a bit drastic holding yourself together, which is one reason why I'm not keen to go out in public just yet – I'm still alive and things are functioning, and the achiness seems to be getting less. I can still put my head down however and go straight to sleep, so obviously need rest.

I was in the middle of just such a sleep about ten this morning when Celia rang. She works for my doctor, so she has access to reports as part of her job. And she rang to say my biopsy results had come through. No sign of cancer. I was so groggy from sleep that I didn't really take it in and had to ring her back to confirm what she'd actually said.

So, whatever's going on in the body with the prostate, it's not the famous big 'C.' Presumably something will still have to be sorted, but that's one negative factor eliminated. That's *real* joy.

Comments:

Katyzzz: You really have been having a rough trot, Mike. Take care and rest up; that's a worthwhile thing to do in the circumstances.

Me: Thanks, Katyzzz. Really appreciate your comments...

God Notes
10 December 2008

Didn't do at all well in hanging onto you or finding any peace or joy in all the kerfuffles over the last few days, Dad. Several times during the evening I was in tears, and struggling greatly to deal with pain—increased by having to wait at A&E, and by anxiety and pressure and so on. Thank you for Celia being there and for her capability, and for good staff at the hospital. But Dad, it really leaves things in a bit of a mess. I'm supposed to play at the St Francis Xavier School's concert tomorrow, and assist with serving food at a friend's wedding on the weekend. There's another friend's concert on Sunday where I'm not only supposed to play the piano, but to prance around doing a silly song as well. Not only am I lacking in energy, the thought of trying to walk much, let alone prance around, is beyond thinking.

Dear Dad, help me to regain some strength and mobility.

A&E is the commonly-used abbreviation for the Accident and Emergency Department of New Zealand hospitals.

St Francis Xavier's is a local primary (elementary) school, and I've played at their annual (now biannual) Christmas musical since one of my sons was around eight or nine, which means I've been doing it for well over twenty years. As I recall, I had to renege on this occasion, and I avoided doing any prancing for the other concert.

God Notes
11 December 2008

Thank you that prostate cancer has been written out of the equation—it's great news, though I'm finding it a bit difficult to appreciate it with the catheter and me not seeing eye to eye (as it were) about how things should be behaving. If this side of things would settle down it would be good. I'm still shuffling along like an old man.

Work Report
11 December, 2008
The Saga Continues: *as you might have expected it would*

By yesterday afternoon, instead of all the urine draining out the catheter, some of it insisted on coming out normally. Well, as normally as possible, since there isn't much room left in the opening of the penis once it has a catheter in there. It would happen quite suddenly, as though I'd left going to the loo for too long and the matter had become urgent.

Wetting pants and floors ain't fun. It might be par for the course for some ninety-year-olds, but I'm still a bit younger than that.

Anyway, I rang the nurse at our health centre and she suggested the catheter might not be fitting correctly, or some other possibility, and in the end I went over there to get her to check it out. It turned out it was lacking a bit of the fluid that keeps the balloon up inside the bladder, but otherwise it was working fairly normally. This, it seems, is a not uncommon problem with catheters.

The urgent need to go to the loo didn't improve, though at least it wasn't happening as fast in the evening as it had in the afternoon. I suspect panic starts to set in at various points, which won't help the issue.

Celia and I debated going back to A&E, but in the end decided to try and get a night's sleep, and the general relaxation that brings. I woke up this morning thinking it would be better to go back to the Urology people rather than the Emergency Department, so I rang them. The Secretary couldn't find much information on me, which was a bit of a surprise, but said she'd contact the Registrar as soon as she could and see what he said.

Apparently he said to go to my doctor, have the catheter removed, see if I could pee properly, and if not, stick it back in again. I rang Celia (she's the office manager/receptionist at the Health Centre, you might remember) and she was very surprised. The GPs don't insert catheters at all, she said. They can take them out, which is easy enough, but certainly don't put them in.

At that point one of the doctors there recommended giving me some tablets that ease the spasm/urgency thing, so that's what I've now got. Just to add to the increasing list of tablets. But at least since I took the first one, things have settled, and I've actually managed to walk around the house and garden without holding myself together.

But the day was not over.

Another woman from Urology rang this afternoon to say she'd got my message "a few minutes before" that I wanted someone to call me. I hadn't rung them a few minutes before, and neither had Celia. Bit of a mystery. I can only conclude that they'd finally got around to answering my original message that I'd left on their voicemail this morning.

Anyway, I explained the situation again, and asked whether it was likely I'd be having an appointment with a Urologist any time soon. She wasn't sure, as there was nothing listed yet. I asked how long I'd need to have the catheter in.

"Six weeks is the norm," she says.

"Six weeks?"

"The body usually needs six weeks to get back to normal and relax."

We discussed this a bit, and the fact that with the Christmas holidays coming up there won't be anyone much around in the department anyway. Finally, feeling rather low, I rang off. My hope now is that since the right hand doesn't seem to know what the left hand is doing at the hospital, including the Urology Department, that someone will ring up tomorrow or Monday and say I've got an appointment to go in and see them. You'd think they'd have some system to stop people falling between the two hands, but if they have, it ain't working.

God Notes
12 December 2008

Dad, things seem to get more complex by the minute. Yesterday someone at Urology—I think it wasn't actually a nurse, and it certainly wasn't a doctor—claimed I'd need to have the catheter in for six weeks, so things could settle down. I'm looking for a second opinion to come through on that, because it's not only rather ridiculous, but it's different by about five weeks to what the A&E doctor said. I'm leaving it to you but also doing a bit of work on my own. In other words, if that really is the truth, I'll hand it over to you and live with it. If it's not, I'd hope to hear from one of the urologists much sooner than that.

Dad, strangely I don't feel particularly anxious about the six weeks thing—it's as though you gave me the gift of not letting it get on top of me at the time I heard about it. I'm still fragile emotionally, but getting more confident in dealing with what's going on—most of the time.

"For I am brought very low," it says in Psalm 79. Thank you, Dad, for your being there when I'm so low—even though I can barely appreciate it.

I certainly have had some very low moments over the last week or so but you keep hauling me up again—thank you, Dad, and thank you especially for Celia who is a gift of great breadth and depth to me.

Work Report
12 December 2008
Six Weeks Reduced

In the last episode of the prostate saga I wrote that someone from the Urology Department had claimed it would be six weeks before I'd get rid of the catheter. On Friday morning, I decided to have another go at seeing whether we could get a bit further with the removal of the thing, on the basis that being strung between four different departments (Urology, Emergency, Day Surgery and my own GP) I might as well see whether someone else in the group had different information.

So I rang the Urology Secretary again. By this time she'd received the notes from Emergency—which was a plus—and I asked if there was any sign of a follow-up appointment to my biopsy. There still wasn't, but she said she'd called the Head of Department and ask him about the situation. This was a different reaction to the one I got from the woman on the previous day, who I think was basically a clerical worker with a smattering of not-necessarily useful knowledge. [*In hindsight this was probably a typical bit of arrogance on my part.*]

The Secretary rang back within a few minutes, which was great, to tell me that I now have an appointment on Thursday, at 8.30 am. Exactly two weeks from the day of the biopsy.

Superb!

I can cope with having this blasted catheter for that short a period. Six weeks would have been really rather frightful. Yes, I know people have much worse suffering than I'm having, but I don't see any point in *wanting* suffering if there's no reason for it.

Meanwhile, because I've been feeling so much better (the urinary tract infection seems to have cleared up) I managed to go to work yesterday for six hours, and coped pretty well. And then in the evening did another two and a half hours of practices for the concert on Sunday, at which I'm now accompanying all the singers. Originally I was supposed to be sharing the playing with someone else, but he got too busy.

Yesterday I was walking around most of the time without too much difficulty. Seems like the catheter and what it's attached to have come to an amicable agreement about how to hang in there. Today it's not quite so settled, but I'm still feeling heaps better, and that in itself is a bonus. No running, leaping, skipping—or prancing—as of this moment, but maybe even that'll be achieved after Thursday!

Work Report
13 December 2008
Imaginative marketing, *or bottomless imagination?*

This has almost nothing to do with the subject of this book. It was a post written between the prostate-focused ones, and makes for a bit of light relief.

I've been talking about areas of the body that I don't normally mention on the blog quite a bit of late, so it's probably not inappropriate to write the following.

Every so often I've had to use suppositories for the rear end to alleviate hemorrhoids and the like. I won't say any more about that, except that in the past the product used for this has been something called Preparation H, which has been around for years.

I went to the pharmacy the other day to buy some and was told it's no longer available. No explanation; it's just gone. So the alternative was a product with the extraordinary name: Anusol. It took me a moment to realize that when you speak the word out loud it sounds like Anus-hole. Good grief.

What marketing manager in the world would have come up with that name? One who doesn't understand English, maybe?

Anyway, I took it back to work and mentioned it to a colleague. She said it's a wonder it's not called Arse-'ole. Apparently, in the first season of the US version of the TV show, *Little Britain*, a group of Anusol executives are having a meeting in which they are being informed that Anusol is being renamed because consumers didn't like the product name. You think? Plainly the executives never had this meeting in real life.

Work Report
15 December, 2008
Roll on Thursday: *only three more sleeps*

I can't wait to get rid of this catheter. The only advantage of it is that I can legitimately use the disability toilet at work—it's closer than the gents and there's a lot more room, something you need when emptying a catheter.

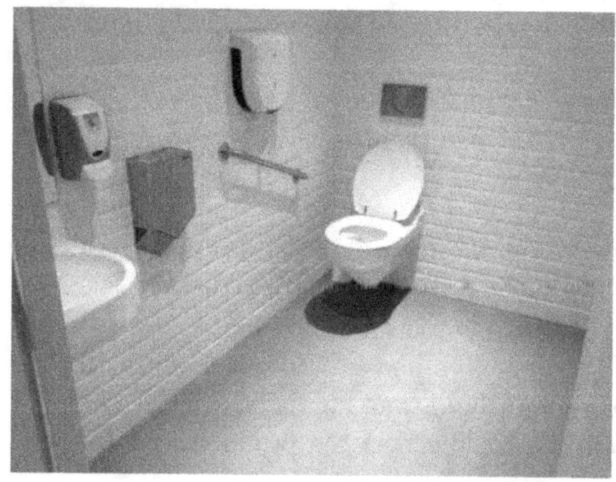

A typical disability toilet—note how much room there is.

I think the most inhibiting thing is not being able to walk quickly. I'm a person who's always walked at a decent speed, which means I also get a bit of decent exercise in the process. Over the last week I've been walking round like an old man who's forgotten where his muscles are.

And the thing makes me tense: I can't tell whether I'm just generally uncomfortable or whether it's tension in my legs that's making me feel unlike my normal self. I find it difficult to get past the fact that when I'm suffering in some way, however small it may be, I feel less like my usual self, because I know what it's like to be well. At the end of last week, after the antibiotics had pretty much done their work, I was feeling quite healthy again, and it was great.

I need to get on and do things that require a bit of energy—otherwise I can see myself having to take fat burners or the like just to keep myself from growing bigger than all my clothes.

But this blasted thing hanging around down below my belt (and I don't mean the one God gave me) is stopping me from real activity—running up or down stairs, striding down the hill to work, zipping across the street avoiding traffic. Just a walk to the library from my office last Friday took me around ten minutes—and it's only a block and a half away.

Roll on Thursday!

During the time I'm writing about in this book, I worked in an office, in a job that wasn't physically very challenging. It occurs to me that dealing with a catheter and a physically-demanding job must be extremely difficult.

Dave has an interesting comment on using disability toilet—at this point he was self-catheterizing, something I'll comment on later:

Dave

I was reflecting the other day on something I need to bear in mind more often than I do. Because of my prostate/plumbing problems, I need to carry a little bit of "apparatus" with me during the day. It is a fine tube or catheter and three to four times a day I am to use it so that I can completely empty my bladder. It is no big deal; it is much better than wearing a permanent catheter and in all other respects life for me is normal. But this gadget has to be washed in warm water and so I need to have a hand basin with hot running water. I also need to carry a tube of KY Jelly; so, as you can imagine, it is better if I have a reasonable measure of privacy. That is easy at home, but at the church or in public toilets it is not always possible.

Sometimes in a public toilet, the washing is a rushed furtive activity with an ear open hoping nobody is going to walk in. In these places, life can be awkward. Because of this whenever I am away from home and using public toilets, I often choose to use the one labeled "Disabled," because it provides a private hand basin. The thing that can be embarrassing is that when you leave or enter the cubicle or toilet labelled 'Disabled,' you sometimes see accusing looks from people who think you have no disability. I once heard one lady say to another, "He doesn't have a wheelchair." Another time when I came out of the disabled toilet a person waiting to use another cubicle commented, "That's a bit cheeky!" as I went past. I sometimes want to yell, "Well, I do have a disability. It is just that you cannot see it!"

God Notes
17 December 2008
Wednesday, *the day before the catheter was due to be removed.*

Dad, I really want to see an end of this catheter tomorrow in the "Trial of Void." Please don't let there be any complications, either from my own nervousness, or from anything physical. Please help me to get back to normality. And, Dad, if there's no cancer with the prostate, what *is* going on? I feel really down about it all just as the moment. Help me to get through today and face tomorrow with peace.

Well, some of these prayers got answered...and some didn't.

Chapter four

My catheter and I have an ongoing relationship, but not a convivial one

Work Report
18 December 2008
No Go: *in and out again*

Back to Day Surgery today for the wonderfully-named exercise: Trial of Void. This, in layman's terms, means being able to empty your bladder successfully after you've had a catheter taken out.

I was as nervous about this as I've ever been about anything, because if I didn't manage the "trial" I'd have had the catheter out for nothing, and would have to have another one put back in.

Part of the joy of the Trial of Void is that you have to drink lots of water while sitting around in the ward doing nothing. I did the Sudoku in the newspaper (no great achievement since it was an Easy one), and tried to read Ian Rankin's appropriately-named *Strip Jack*, but neither of these held my attention as much as the voiding.

The voiding went okay at first. The male nurse had lined up half-a-dozen urine bottles, and every time I went to the toilet I was supposed to fill one of these—not literally fill, but make a decent attempt—and hand it back to him to measure. An exciting job for the nurse.

The first two tries were okay, though not outstanding; by the time I got to the third things were starting to seize up again, and only a little dribble appeared. Eventually it got to that same ridiculous point where I was desperate to go, but nothing would work.

Which meant back to a catheter again.

I was pretty distressed about this, and pretty fed up too. But as both the nurse and the doctor who came to put the catheter back in said, it wasn't the fact that I was tensed up that was causing the problem; rather the prostate is squeezing the life out of the urethra even though the latter is only trying to do its job. It's what happens when the prostate gets too big for its boots.

So I was in Day Surgery from 8.30 am till at least 1.30 pm. Missed the work luncheon—couldn't have eaten anything anyway—and eventually came home and rested after the ordeal.

I ought to feel thoroughly unhappy, but the strange thing is that I don't. Having got used to the idea of wearing a catheter over the last eight days, having another one doesn't seem to be quite such a big deal. Perhaps it's fitting a bit better; certainly it doesn't feel as though it's cutting into me all the time. And another plus is knowing that having the thing there means I won't have any difficulties with emptying my bladder.

Of course, it's still a nuisance: cleaning it up, and adding a night bag when you go to bed, all takes up time that would be better used in doing something more interesting. But the goal seems more in sight. I have another appointment due in a fortnight, which being New Year's Day will no doubt get delayed until the following week. And at the appointment I actually get to see the Urologist.

It looks as though some operation will have to take place, possibly the one where they scrape out the inner area of the prostate so that the urethra has some room to breathe. Hopefully not the one where they remove the prostate completely.

Time will tell.

God Notes
20 December 2008

Dad, I now have to live with the catheter until 13 January, at the very least, and probably longer. Can't see them taking it out just at the moment, particularly after the kerfuffle on Thursday. It's sometimes quite painful in the way it rubs on the opening to my penis. I'll have to find a way to alleviate that in some measure; that's the worst thing about it. If I can get that sorted I can probably cope, even though it's rather restrictive.

Dad, I need your peace during this time—certainly you've helped me in a good measure since the catheter went back in, but twenty-four days before anything else happens seems a long time.

My pains are vastly less than those that my friend with breast cancer has been going through, so help me to remember this when I get uptight about the whole thing. I can endure it. It's not "normal" but it isn't way off the scale. Dad, let there be some outcome from the January 13 visit, so I can see how long I'm having to wait and can know what's ahead a bit more. Keep me healthy otherwise.

Thank you that I already got "moved up" the list because someone cancelled. Just keep your eye on things as we progress, please.

When we see that you're just as willing to endure the hard times as to enjoy the good times, we know you're going to make it, no doubt about it. [2 Corinthians 1:7 *The Message*]

Work Report
21 December, 2008
Living with the Catheter again

Got an appointment the day after my Trial of Void (sounds like something judicial) and it isn't till 13 January. As of today, that's twenty-three sleeps by my reckoning.

And, of course, since it's only a visit to the Urologist, it's unlikely anything will be happening with the catheter. So unless someone else gets in on the act, and decides another try at voiding is possible, it looks like I've got the bloomin' thing for the duration.

Friday was a horrible day: I couldn't get comfortable with the catheter, no matter how I tried. I was at work, struggling to sit comfortably. Had an agonizing walk when I went to meet a friend of mine at lunchtime, and probably looked like death-warmed-up when I arrived at the café where we meet.

Meanwhile, the District Nurse had dropped off some "supplies" at home, amongst which was a kind of band that holds the catheter more firmly on the upper thigh. After a bit of working out of the placement of it with Celia—no room for embarrassment in our house at the moment—I found that I could get much more comfortable, and yesterday and today have been turning points. I'm much more mobile too: getting up and down out of chairs is easier, I've been on the treadmill twice and did a couple of kilometers each time, and am even considering walking to work tomorrow. This is major progress. If I can achieve some exercise, I can cope with the irritations of having the thing.

Mentioning the band that the District Nurse had dropped off makes it sound as though I didn't have anything holding the catheter in place before this. Celia assures me that this couldn't have been the case. We must have devised some alternative of our own until the proper band arrived, or else had some inferior strap.

What I only appear to have mentioned in passing is something that initially was quite concerning. Whenever I went to the toilet for a bowel motion (or, as they call it in medical parlance, an "evacuation") the contractions would force urine out past *the catheter, and a small amount of it would squeeze out of the penis. Once I found out this was "normal" I accepted it was just another facet of wearing a catheter. However, it was always accompanied by short but considerable pain, as though something was being torn inside the penis.*

And on those occasions when I had blockage problems with the catheter, the times when things were so bad I had to visit A&E, urine would ooze out through the penis instead of the catheter. This was very unpleasant, and increasingly painful. Obviously the bladder and the catheter between them decided that neither was giving way, and the urine would build up fearsomely in the bladder itself.

God Notes
23 December 2008

Dad, thank you that I'm able to walk and move more freely, and that I'm not finding the thing quite so inhibiting. But I'm still dropping into low patches and that's upsetting Celia. Help me to overcome those too, and rejoice in the midst of all this.

The Journal
26 December 2008

Wearing the catheter is just bloody painful some days, especially when the underside of the tip of the penis gets made raw by the rubbing of the catheter on it. For the past week things haven't been too bad in that respect, as between us, Celia and I worked out how to keep it from moving unnecessarily. But yesterday when we were helping at the Christmas Dinner at the Church of Christ, for some reason the catheter began cutting into me again. Believe it or not, the pain is debilitating. I wind up feeling quite exhausted from it. And, of course, I immediately feel restricted in movement.

Anyway, I had a longish bath last night, and daubed a pile of Vaseline on the penis tip, and things have been much better today. The Vaseline makes a great difference. It's extraordinary stuff.

What I'm struggling with is the possibility of not being able to live without the catheter. Going back to normality seems a million miles away. It's stupid, but I'm having to work hard not to go into the beginnings of a kind of panic whenever I think about it. I only need to see some guy on TV walking normally or doing something perfectly usual, and it triggers off something in my brain: *you won't be able to do that again.* It's like the kind of panic that used to come when I'd see ads for other shop's sales when I was running the bookstore, and I'd know that we could never compete with their promotional budget.

The reality of course is that I will get rid of this thing, and that the plumbing will come back to normality. *When* is the question.

What I need to remember is that after the time when I had the catheter in and out (the day of the biopsy) I was fine until I got the urinary tract infection. That was what set things off again. In the days between that and the biopsy I'd been as fit as a fiddle. So blame it all on the UTI (as opposed to blaming it on the Bossa Nova).

42

More importantly, somehow I've got to get past the fear of a non-normal future. I guess it happens to anyone who finds themselves in a situation where things aren't functioning properly. Certainly some people don't get back to normality; but plenty do, and I need to see that as the way ahead, rather than this current situation.

Yesterday at the Christmas Dinner, I stood serving potatoes beside a lawyer who used to come into the secondhand bookshop that was situated inside the Christian bookshop I managed. He'd buy books regularly. He told me yesterday that he'd had cancer—the bladder, urinary tract and so on had all been affected, and now he wears a colostomy bag all the time. Don't ask me how we got into that conversation amongst the potatoes, but compared to that, a catheter seems child's play. I should be grateful that I don't have cancer in the prostate (and presumably don't have it anywhere else) and that I'm reasonably fit and healthy other than whatever's going on with the bladder, and that even that may well come back to some sort of normality in due course. At the moment, the worst I'm looking at is a scraping out of the inside of the prostate. Doesn't sound pleasant, but presumably it can be lived through—a musician friend of mine has had it done, for example, and he's functioning normally.

Work Report
29 December 2008
PUBS: ***The Color Purple***

The following may not be for the squeamish.

Further to my ongoing business of having to wear a catheter, I had an interesting experience today.

Wearing one of these things requires you to empty it regularly, as you'd expect, so you get used to the color of what's being emptied. It's usually pretty similar to what you'd excrete if you weren't using a catheter .

Anyway, at about eleven this morning, I went to empty it and discovered a good deal of reddish color in the urine. My first reaction was probably what most people's would be: I'm bleeding somewhere inside.

Worse, just before lunch I emptied it out again only to find that the color was now purple—not bright purple, but definitely purple. I went to lunch with a friend feeling more than a little distracted.

When I got back to work, however, the color had reverted to normal, and there was no sign of anything discoloring it at all. Googled it. As one does.

"Purple urine" was sufficient to get an explanation. It's officially called Purple Urine Bag Syndrome. Seems reasonable enough. According to one site:

Purple urine bag syndrome—shortened, as you'd expect by now, to PUBS—*is a rare syndrome associated with alkaline urine and some urinary tract infections, and is more frequently observed in chronically catheterized and constipated women.*

Note that use of the word "rare." More on this later. Anyway, even though I wasn't a chronically cathetized and constipated woman, PUBS had occurred. So some bacteria must have got itself mixed in somewhere.

This happens because the catheter itself changes the normal color associated with pee (anything from clear to dirty brown) to red or blue, violet or purple. Good to have a choice. The color can depend on the tube it's running through, or the bag itself. The cause is still being debated by those investigating it but generally it's thought that one of the amino acids in your system—tryptophan, in this instance—is affected by, or reacts to, particular bacteria in the gut.

What happens then gets a bit too scientific for me to put easily into layman's language; suffice to say the bacterial mix gets absorbed into the delightfully named "portal circulation"— small blood vessels leading into bigger ones—and then there's another chemical reaction in the liver. This comes after a series of "detoxification transformations"—another great phrase— which basically just means that any nasty stuff is cleaned out.

Okay, without understanding everything there, I got the drift. Another site put it more simply: The color is seen when the pink-red pigment indirubin or its cousin, indigo blue, interact with the plastic of the catheter or urine bag.

So it wasn't just me—the bag was partly to blame.

As it happened, I was talking to the District Nurse later in the afternoon, and I mentioned the color change. Obviously PUBS isn't as rare as the website makes out, as she wasn't in the least bit fazed by it. She made it sound as though it happened to most of her cathetized patients at some point!

For a couple of hours around lunch time I was feeling pretty low. I'm good at thanking the Lord when things have come right, but not so good at trusting Him in the middle of unpleasant surprises.

God Notes
31 December 2008

Dad, I don't know why things are manageable one day and so uncomfortable the next. After an increasingly sore time yesterday, I felt really low last night, in tears, and hopeless. Dad, thank you for Celia's practical nature.

Restore my hope. More than that, give me hope. I don't appear to have much at the moment. Celia's still talking about going camping in the holidays, which just sounds like adding complications galore to my situation.

Getting to sound like a real whine bag about this point, especially when I consider that while I was putting this book together I discovered that some men (and some women) have to self-catheterize on a daily basis. In fact a friend emailed me and said he had to do it four times a day. People who self-catheterize have to be trained to do it, and it may be done up to six times a day. And yes, it still involves putting a catheter tube up inside your penis.

God Notes
4 January 2009

Since I last wrote the feeling of hopelessness hasn't been so evident, and even though we've had some real frazzly moments, with the catheter tube separating in the night—and during the day!—I'm generally better. Yesterday, things were uncomfortable, more from the spasm type of angle. Whether it was because the tube kept coming loose or what, I don't know. Anyway, here we are, and thank you for another day.

Dad, you've kept me through thick and thin over many years; you've blessed my life in immeasurable ways. There's no reason why I should be blessed when so many others aren't. Help me to remember this when I complain or get upset, as I seem to do so easily with the stuff that's going on. It's the feeling of not being in control, I guess. Help me to remember, when I get most distressed, that *you* are in control, however little I may sense that.

Work Report
4 January, 2009
Genes and Prostate Cancer: *not the last word*

Back in September 2007 I wrote a piece called *Good News on the Prostate Front*. [This is reprinted in this book as the second item in the Extras section because it's sometimes hard to find online.] The article should probably have been entitled *Mostly Good News on the Prostate Front* because, in fact, even though there's now a test available that's more accurate than the biopsy one that's presently done, this test is only telling us that there's a possibility of prostate cancer in later life. It doesn't actually tell you how you're going to avoid it.

The test is a genetic one and identifies five gene markers for hereditary prostate cancer. So far so good. You can get the test done at any stage of your manhood, long before the PSA might be showing up some negative signs.

But the question is: what next? All this test is telling you is that you may be likely to get prostate cancer. Or not. If you *are* likely to get it, what can you do about it?

Well, the short answer is, Not a lot.

There are any number of articles on the Net with "answers" for avoiding prostate cancer. They follow a pattern: drink lots of water, avoid excess alcohol, keep your weight under control, and eat tomatoes because they contain Lycopene. Lycopene is an antioxidant compound that gives tomatoes and certain other fruits and vegetables their color; it's supposed to help you avoid the cancer. Eat carrots, and, last but not least, maintain a good mental attitude.

Dare I say, Oh, puleeese! Without sounding like a know-it-all, I don't think any of these are necessarily going to stop the possibility of cancer. I continue to eat tomatoes and carrots as I've always done. I drink water, I don't particularly drink alcohol (just because I never have). My weight isn't quite at the right place it should be, but I'm not carrying a lot of it—and I've always walked a good deal.

As for mental attitude, this is one of those non-scientific approaches on the fringes of medicine which haven't yet been confirmed as having particular value. Most of us would love to have a continuously positive mental attitude, but it doesn't necessarily come easily. We can't always avoid anger, stress, even depression. Some of these things we just have to live with and sort out the best we can.

My biopsy showed I didn't have cancer, but what if it had shown that I did? Would all that walking, tomato and carrot-eating, etc have actually proved anything? Could I crow about my "good" behavior? I doubt it. If anything, I was fortunate, lucky, blessed—whatever.

A good friend of mine developed breast cancer last year. She'd always eaten healthy food—almost to the point of obsession. The connection isn't proven, is all I can say.

Of course it's better to be eating good stuff, exercising, and generally avoiding unhealthy emotions. It's also a fact of life that we live in a world where nothing is perfect in terms of health.

Incidentally, the gene test isn't readily available from your GP as yet. Or from anyone else. It's coming, but you may still have to wait a while.

In the fourth section of Extras there are a couple more posts on this topic. Since beginning to write this book I've come across a group online called Pints for Prostates whose motto is "reaching men through the universal language of beer." I'm not sure what they think of the "avoid excess alcohol" approach to avoiding prostate cancer. You can find their website in the "Links of interest" section.

God Notes
5 January 2009

Dad, I'm generally more relaxed about things—only eight more days to go till the urology appointment—not sure what will be happening from there. Let it be something "definite" at least, and help me to be at peace about whatever it is, rather than anxious.

Work Report
5 January, 2009
Repeating the Process: *highs and lows*

I got up yesterday morning, felt good, walked to work for the first time in a while (partly because of all the Christmas holidays) and then, as the day went on, things got very uncomfortable, with lots of stinging as the catheter affected a certain important part of my male anatomy.

Felt exhausted when I got home, had a bit of a kip, and then later on did the vacuuming. I was going to go in the bath after that, to try and soothe things down below, but then had one of those moments when I just had to pee, and instead of it going down the catheter it came out as normal. (Quite a nice feeling, in a way, but not what you want as things stand at present.)

This was concerning, as it shouldn't happen, so we rang A&E to see if they had a nurse who could just check the water levels in the balloon that holds the catheter in place inside my bladder. Nope. They were expecting lots of people as a result of a big accident, so I'd be way down on the priority list.

So Celia, quick-thinking as ever, rang one of the nurses who works in the same health centre. And the nurse offered to go up to the centre and check out the catheter for me. What generosity!

She found that the water level was about four milliliters (about a teaspoon) short—it should have ten milliliters in total. This is why things had become particularly irritating during the day. But the process of correcting this was extremely unpleasant, particularly as no anesthetic was involved.

This morning I got up, feeling shivery and very much under the weather, as though I'd dropped into a hole. Finally, though both of us were running late for work, Celia took a urine sample from the catheter (a bit of a mission in itself) and I went over with her to the health centre. The nurse "dipsticked" it (used a urine test strip coated with various chemicals which react to bacteria) and pronounced it full of bugs. Obviously it'll get properly tested today at the lab, but the dipstick approach is enough to go on.

So it was back to the doctor and back onto antibiotics and here I am at home not allowed to go to work today. I've never had so much time off work in my life! [*Fortunately at this point in my career I was working in a place where flexi-time was the norm.*]

Comments:
Bevetal: What a pain...all this time off, and not well enough to enjoy it ! Hope you're more comfortable soon.

Me: I'm feeling more comfortable at the moment, but the energy levels ain't high!

Bacteria is very common with catheters that stay in for more than two or three weeks. Antibiotics will work, but the bugs get tougher and stronger and can form a kind of colony, making them difficult to treat. The real preference is not to have a catheter in for too long altogether, but sometimes this isn't practical.

God Notes
6 January 2009

When my anxious thoughts multiply within me, your consolations delight my soul. [Psalm 94:19 - New American Standard Bible]

My anxious thoughts are making me more anxious. And worse, Celia's got to the point of having had enough of it all. I can understand that—it drags you down and you feel as though you can't lift the other person's spirit, let alone your own. Help me, Dad, I'm really struggling. Please give me some ease of heart, some peace. Let your consolations comfort me and delight me. Let me have courage, which I've always lacked.

The Journal
8 January 2009

Some of the things that haven't made it into the blog regarding the famous catheter:

Last night, at some small hour, I was awake and trying to get comfortable (erections and catheters don't mix) when I felt a fluttering on my leg. I thought it must have been the tube wriggling, but then I felt the same thing on the other leg. Had a horrible sensation that it might be something in the bed besides the tube, so I felt around—cautiously—with my hand. The flickering happened again. I got out of bed as fast as I could, saying to Celia, "There's something in the bed!" She thought I was having a hallucination but she still got out to investigate. At first we couldn't see anything. And then a moth flew out of my shorts, where it had obviously gone to hide from all the fuss.

Another night I woke up feeling I'd wet myself—which shouldn't have been possible. Nope, possible all right. The tube between the internal part of the catheter and the bit where it joins onto the day bag had come loose, and there was a sudden backflow up the pipe. This delightful experience happened at least twice in the daytime as well, and would have gone on, presumably, except that I sealed up the joint with several sticking plasters.

And the other night, one of those nights when everything seems to be loading on top of you, I had a nose bleed just as I was trying to get organized for bed. It's tricky enough getting clothes off and pajamas on over the catheter bag at the best of times, but when your nose is dripping as well, it becomes a major undertaking.

Walking with the catheter even partly full is like wading on one leg through the sea. There's this unpleasant sloshing sound, which you're sure everyone else can hear. [*My cousin, who's currently in the same predicament, says it feels like his leg's swollen.*] And getting it to sit where it's comfortable is a major undertaking too. When I first got it, I just had it hanging fairly loose—until I realized how painful that could be. Later on, I used the leg strap with a little Velcro hook on it which you can fit the tube through. Using this on alternate legs for several days was fine, and I could get round mostly fairly comfortably. But on Monday, after having walked down the hill to work, the pulling on my penis got sharper and sharper, and by the time I got home that night I was exhausted. Turned out I had another blasted infection!

Curiously enough, when I went to see the doctor about this on Tuesday morning, and I was getting dressed again after she inspected things, I tucked the tube up inside my pants into the crotch area—as much as I could—and discovered that it sat there perfectly well of its own accord. So that's the current modus operandi. No doubt it'll change again at some point!

Here's another view on living with a catheter, from Dave. He had an enlarged prostate like me, but he had two biopsies to my one. This post dates from 15 October 2012.

Dave

On Saturday, I found myself depressed with my "catheter and bag" situation. It felt like my active life had come to an end. Here were the changes I had encountered. A week before, my wife and I had made love, but now that was impossible and there is a possibility it may never happen again. A week before, I could run, ride my bike, and play energetic, fast-paced table tennis. This weekend I would not be able to run, riding the bike with a catheter is not advised, and when I played a gentle game of table tennis, I doubled over in pain from a spasm it brought on. Even lifting tables during the week had brought about blood in my urine. So on Saturday I was feeling down. My active life seemed over, and I felt like I may as well pack up, get fat and old, and "wait for God."

I understand exactly what Dave is saying here. There are times in this process when hope flies out the open window. However, something good flew into my window the day after my last journal entry.

Chapter five

Finding out what kind of an operation I'm going to have —

...and a brief holiday before the great event.

Work Report
9 January 2009
And so it goes: *one less sleep*

I've just had a couple of responses to an email I sent out to the wider family a week or so ago, in which I gave some details of our household experiences in 2008, in particular, the current state of health of yours truly.

It was interesting that one of the recipients commented: *Hope you are fully fit and well again...seems like you were never anything else.* That's exactly what it's been like. I've rarely had anything more serious than the flu; never had any broken bones, and only a couple of instances where they've had to stitch me up. Even those were fairly minor. Compare this to one of my sons, who, when he was about seven or eight, had four lots of stitches within six months.

Well, the health- debt-collection agency is certainly cashing in over these last few months, one might say. I can't remember whether I wrote about the week of nosebleeds I had, and the double lot of cauterization, which occurred in July last year. I've always had nosebleeds—they run in the family—but never a week's worth. And then there's been all this other prostate stuff.

I was off work again this Tuesday, as I mentioned in the last post, and on both Wednesday and Thursday mornings I seemed

52

fine when I got up. But then I felt lousy within an hour or so. A short nap at work seemed to restore things, so I don't know what was going on in the system. Haven't exactly been working at full strength lately, but at least I've been working. Fortunately it's a quiet time of year.

Today, however, I finished work for three weeks. I'm on leave. Yay!

And I got a call from the Urology Clinic. They've had to cancel all Tuesday afternoon's appointments due to a bereavement, but they're able to see me on Monday morning first thing. So that's good news. One less sleep…

Today I had a long chat with the nurse at the Health Centre who had very obligingly come after hours on Monday evening and sorted me out. I'd already suspected that the Urology appointment wouldn't mean the end of the catheter; it's more likely to be about a plan of attack regarding the prostate itself. The nurse said it's likely they'll leave it in for at least another couple of weeks, and then do another trial of void. Apparently it's the only way they can check to see whether the bladder has settled down and whether the muscles have decided they cope with normal life again.

I'd already pretty much anticipated this, so it wasn't really a surprise. Somehow or other I need to get into the mental state, however, to be able to cope with going through another trial of void (which was definitely a trial last time) and coming out with things functioning. The nurse said that part of the problem is that the biopsy itself can cause swelling of the bladder (which means it retains more liquid) and then the sphincter muscles get themselves out of kilter, and so the process goes.

At least that means it wasn't just my own uptightness at the time of the biopsy that caused the water retention. You might say it was my body going on strike as a result of the invasion.

God Notes
12 January 2009

Dad, urology appointment today. Thank you for it coming a day earlier than expected, and thank you that this morning I'm not feeling so edgy as I was at times yesterday. Help me to cope with whatever is the outcome of today's meeting, especially if it's something worse than I've expected.

Work Report
12 January 2009
The End in Sight: *ever hopeful*

Down to the Urology Department at the hospital today.

Took my Whānau* with me (Celia, in other words), mostly for moral support, but also to ask questions, and to clarify things I'd missed.

Saw yet another doctor (as you'd expect) but he was well-informed, and friendly, and helpful. He had all my notes with him, and got me to "walk through" the process so far, so that we were "on the same page." (It's cliché day; my clichés, not his.) Plenty of time to look at where things have been and what's happened up to this point, so it was all very useful. It was also useful to have it confirmed again that it isn't anything I've done that's caused the water retention problems (and hence the wearing of the catheter). "Nothing you can do can make your bladder stop working," he reiterated.

After the initial discussions, and some confirmatory consultation with his boss, he said there were two options: TORC or TURP. TORC is what I've already had done once—the trial removal of the catheter. He suggested that he put me on Hytrin for a few days beforehand and then see how we went with another removal. I said, "But I've been on Hytrin for several years." This rather puzzled him. "Do you mean for blood pressure?" "No," I said, "for the prostate." Seems like this wasn't quite the norm, although I'm under the impression Hytrin is definitely used for problems resulting from prostate enlargement.

"Well, that only leaves the other option," he said, "as another TORC would achieve nothing."

So it's option number two: TURP. TURP stands for transurethral resection of the prostate, but it means what I thought would be the *only* option: going up through the urethra and scraping out the inside of the prostate so that the urethra can get on and do its job. And relieve itself of wearing a catheter. If

54

you're interested in the device that does it, check out the photo below. Otherwise, move quickly past it.

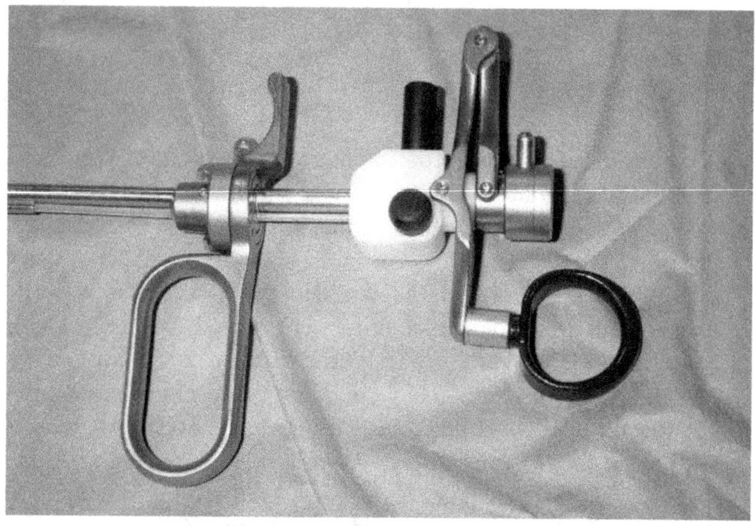

Transurethral Resectoscope.

Note that the photographer has avoided showing us the bit
that does the job.

The urologist explained how it's done, but I didn't ask him for too many details (I've given the basic outline at the end of this post**). I already knew enough to keep me going. Seemingly, the urethra wall and the prostate's exterior are virtually the same thing just below the bladder, which is why the surgeon doesn't have to do any cutting of the urethra itself to achieve the job.

As for when the op is going to be done, I've been put on the "urgent list" because they don't want to keep the catheter in longer than necessary (constant risk of infection) and because they can't do another trial of void. Urgent may not mean tomorrow, but it will mean I'll be up for any cancellations, and should see the thing done in a couple of months at the outside.

At the moment I can't actually imagine it being done to *me*. I was reading the TV review page in the latest NZ Listener on the way home. The writer was talking about a documentary in which someone went with the British soldiers to Afghanistan, as part of their tour of duty. They kept saying they "were putting that to the back of their mind." Think that's the attitude I'll have to take with this as well.

** Whānau is a Māori word meaning immediate and extended family, but it can also extend to spiritual and emotional connections, such as close friends. Already a "multi-layered, flexible and dynamic" word (according to the Encyclopedia of New Zealand)it's been taken over into New Zealand English where it's sometimes used in a typically Kiwi joking sense, so that it includes people who aren't part of your immediate family.*

***For those who want a bit more detail about how the resectoscope works, there's a long thin metal tube that's pushed up inside the urethra. The tube contains a light, a camera, and a loop of wire. The light and camera help the surgeon find the prostate. An electric current heats the loop, and this heated wire is used to cut away the unwanted prostate material. This material collects in the bladder, and is flushed away by the catheter that's inserted after the prostate has been dealt with.*

God Notes
13 January 2009

Dad, yesterday was a great step forward. I feel psychologically a lot better because I have the sense I'm now on the road to recovery, even though I still have the operation ahead. The fact that the operation should sort out the bladder problems, and that I don't have to have another trial of void, is a great plus. As well, yesterday I had very little irritation with the catheter—great all round. Thank you!

The Journal
14 January 2009

Wednesday.
Life with the catheter goes on, and will until the operation to remove the inner part of the prostate is done. Somehow or other I've disassociated myself from what will actually happen on that

day; guess it's too unpleasant to really think about. I know what will happen, pretty much, just don't want to contemplate it.

Earlier I talked about walking while wearing the catheter. It seems there's no one solution to keeping it strapped, or tucked in, or whatever. It won't remain comfortable for more than a few days. The tucked-in approach stopped being comfortable, and I'm back to strapping it. The last three days haven't been too bad at all in that regard. And I've finally stopped wearing a pair of large underpants inside my pajamas at night (started that because we weren't sure how much leaking and other stuff was likely to go on, and because they were much less constricting than my own pants). There's a nice sense of freedom again, which is pleasant. Well, given that I still have the catheter.

I've got a certain freedom in my head as well: knowing that the thing will eventually be sorted is a major plus, something to really look forward to. Far more than the trial of void approach, where you may or may not come out successful.

At this point in the original journal entry I made some comments about sexual matters—and catheters. They were a bit too private to repeat in full here, but suffice to say, intercourse is obviously impossible, even though erections still occur—an uncomfortable process with a catheter. There's not much incentive for intimacy anyway when you're worn out from the drag of carting an extra appendage around all day, or have the day bag connected to the night bag (isn't there a song about that?), the latter hanging out of the bed like a dead weight.

Work Report
16 January 2009
External Plumbing: *bit of a drip*

I went to town on the bus around lunch-time today and noticed when I got to my stop that my left foot seemed to be just a little damp—just below where the nozzle of the catheter bag comes out. Thought it might have been a bit of a drip and didn't give it much attention, but while I was having lunch with a friend, I could feel my left foot getting more and more damp.

Finally went off to the loo to check and found that the nozzle had definitely been leaking onto my foot.

Unfortunately I had to go and see someone else before I could go home and tidy things up, which meant dealing with a very wet sock on that side. I discovered later that the shunt wasn't quite shutting: it needed an additional click to get it to close off completely, though this is the first time it's been a problem.

Ah, the joys of catheters! This isn't the first time one of them has given me a sudden wet surprise.

It'll be good to get back to having to deal only with plumbing on the inside of the body again.

During this next period we went on holiday, firstly at Otematata and then in Cromwell. The Work Report *blog wasn't used during this time, but there are a couple of mentions of problems in my* Travel Diary *blog which I briefly resurrected for the occasion. Otematata is a town that was originally built to house men working on the Benmore Dam. It's now mostly used by holidaymakers. In Cromwell, the old historic part of the town was buried under millions of tons of water as part of a hydro dam project near a town further down the river. Prior to the flooding it was a place where many people went for their holidays, and it also boasted a substantial number of orchards. It now has many permanent residents, vast numbers of holidaymakers, and, along with new orchards, increasing numbers of vineyards.*

God Notes
19 January 2009
In Otematata

Dad, another one of those weeping sessions this morning, of which there have been a few since the catheter arrived. Today, it might partly have been that I slept very badly, being worried that something leakage-wise might happen while using someone else's bed. Partly, I think it's the tension of not knowing when all this will come to an end—and partly it's my concerns about the op itself. Dad, I guess it's also just pent-up stuff. I know it upsets Celia and I feel helpless and hopeless when it's going on. Have no idea how to deal with it. Feel as though you aren't around in relation to it either, even though that's not the truth. Help me, Dad; so many other of our friends go through far worse stuff and are seemingly a lot better at handling it. This is comparatively minor.

Mike Crowl's Travel Diary
19 January 2009
First Day in Otematata

We discovered last night that we weren't supposed to be drinking the water straight out of the tap in the house we're staying in. We discovered this after I'd already had at least two glasses of it with my various tablets. Should have boiled it first.

Found it hard to get to sleep, again: probably felt neurotic about the possibility of adding yet another thing to my current state of health—bacteria from the water. In fact I seem to be all right. I'm finding I'm having occasional really blue days—today started off that way but I'll just have to keep moving forward. How people who have much worse operations to look forward to cope I'm really not sure. I'm having enough trouble with this relatively minor one.

Mike Crowl's Travel Diary
20 January 2009
Second Day

Neither of us has been laid low by drinking untreated water, so obviously our stomachs are tougher than the Waitaki District Council believes. Which is a good thing. However, today we got a call from my doctor saying that she'd written out a script for yet another antibiotic. I've already got enough tablets of a different kind to last me till next week, but it seems that on the basis of the lab results that came back after my last urine sample, (taken when I visited the After Hours doctor last Friday night for yet another issue with the catheter), they think I need to be on this different antibiotic. Will I be resistant to anything at the end of all this?

Anyway, to get this script filled we had to go to the nearest chemist which is in Twizel, a good half hour up the road from

Otematata. Celia found this out from a woman who lives near where we're staying. The woman said there was a bit of a shortcut to Twizel on the Omarama Rd at Prohibition Rd. (Interesting name for a road.)

The Journal
22 January 2009
In Cromwell

Yesterday was a strange day. I started out all right with the catheter, being quite comfortable. However within a short time it was pulling at me something awful, and I was getting that jabbing inside my penis I've had on other occasions, including, most recently, the night we went down to After Hours. (I haven't mentioned the After Hours visit previously because it was just more of the same old cleaning out the catheter stuff.)

While we were still in Otematata, a nurse from After Hours rang on the cellphone and said the doctor had prescribed some tablets for thrush as well, because that had shown up in my urine sample. That would be what was causing the occasional itching, although itching has been the least of my problems. Anyway, we asked her to send the prescription through to Twizel again, and said we'd go and pick it up—not having anything else in particular to do, and it meant we'd get out of the house for a while.

While I was at Twizel I could hardly walk—don't know whether it was that the catheter was sitting funny or something, so I tried some adjusting, and when we got home to Otematata everything came right again. Weird. If only it would stay consistent, it would help a lot. Before we had tea we went for a walk along by the dam again, and I was pretty much up to normal speed, apart from watching out for stones that might cause any jarring if I stepped on them.

It seems to be that the body has a great deal of inbuilt shock absorbing: but with this catheter in place, that absorbing is nowhere near as effective. It comes as something of a surprise to realize just how much the groin and loin area of your body acts as a fulcrum, and just how strong the muscles down there must be in terms of assisting with lifting and general movement. With them less than mobile, everything else seems under par.

The Journal
23 January 2009
In Cromwell

Celia went for a swim this afternoon, but I'm not really fussed about trying to wrap up the catheter's tubing and bag underneath my swimming togs. It might be manageable, but as of today I haven't seen it as an option. I'm not sure what other people would think I was carrying inside my trunks.

She also made some comments somewhere along the line— last night I think, after I'd had a day of soreness, and had been going on and on about it—that I need to be positive about where things are going. And having some optimism *is* necessary: it's healthy, quite apart from getting my mind off the problems. It's what I said I'd do late last year, when I listed out in the blog the things I wanted this year to be about, rather than being all about the prostate. At that stage, of course, I hadn't had the biopsy and all its subsequent problems. It's interesting to speculate that if I hadn't had the biopsy whether I'd have had any of the problems I'm having. The trauma seems to have set things like the water retention and the urinary infections off. At that time I thought I wasn't even having problems peeing, unlike many prostate problem sufferers, but in hindsight this wasn't true, as I noted in a post about the biopsy.

Of course, we don't know whether these things may have come about anyway, but it would be nice to think that they wouldn't have. And without the biopsy, of course, we'd have no assurance on the cancer side, so I suppose that has to be weighed up against the issues I've got just now.

I must say I've struggled to keep optimistic since the catheter went in. I was far more positive immediately after the biopsy day than I have been since. I guess the issue to a great extent is that I've never really had any physical handicap of any sort for more than a few days. Last Tuesday made six weeks of living with the catheter—when I first heard that I might have it that long I was very concerned. (I met an old friend in town one day who cheerfully told me he'd had his in for three months.) The six weeks haven't exactly flown, but I'm still alive. I've suffered a lot of relatively minor inconvenience, even if at times it can be the equivalent of someone poking a knife up under your fingernail at regular intervals. I've gotten depressed about it, but have come up again more than once. The good days have been fine, the difficult days get left behind like any other days.

The Journal
25 January 2009
In Cromwell

Woke up from a very deep sleep about 1.30 am last night to find that somehow or other the bed around my right foot was soaked. It seems that the day bag wasn't draining into the night bag and consequently once it got fairly full it just pushed the urine out. Plus I think I might have had my leg on top of it. A very unpleasant feeling to wake up to, especially in a motel bed. Fortunately we'd bought a piece of waterproof material, so that at least stopped the bed getting wet. But the undersheet had a large wet patch on it, and some of the upper sheet was wet too.

Work Report
26 January 2009
Staying Positive: ***cranberry juice***

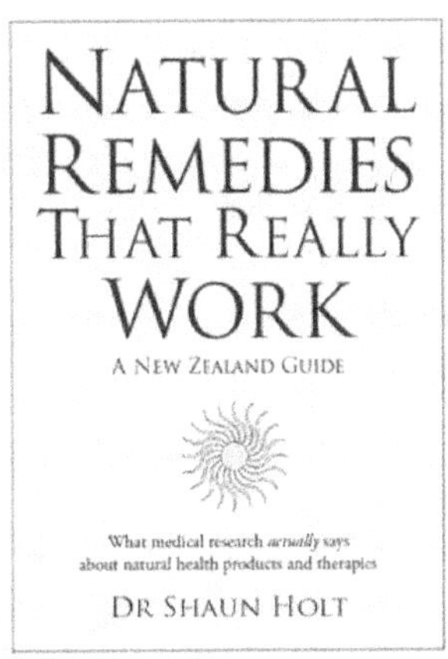

While we were in the Cromwell Pharmacy last week, I noticed a book on the counter, *Natural Remedies That Really Work* by Dr Shaun Holt, and on looking through it saw that it was recommending cranberry juice for urinary tract infections, something that I'd already had recommended to me by a friend I've met through work.

The book looked interesting and seemed to weave a decent path between the extremes of believing everything about health remedies and believing nothing. The pharmacist said she'd bought the copy from PaperPlus, just across the mall, so I went over and asked if they had it. The young lady gave me the impression that serving customers wasn't really what she was there for, particularly when she couldn't find the book on her computer—I'd given her the title slightly wrongly. I suggested we do the old-fashioned thing and look on the shelf—a suggestion which didn't seem to amuse her—and so we did, and there it was.

Obviously with all these "natural" remedies you've got to be careful that you're not working against the medicines you're getting from other sources, but I don't think extra help, in the way of cranberry, will do any harm. Last week I was having to have eight capsules a day for thrush as well as the other tablets I'm already taking. I'll start rattling soon.

On pages 109-110 of the book, there are the following questions in relation to staying positive when your health is under par:

- *What can I do to achieve the best possible outcomes?*
- *What are innovative responses to the situation?*
- *What do I need to know to reach a productive conclusion?*
- *What can I learn from this situation that will help me in the future?*
- *What is an interpretation of this event that will motivate me to continue to strive for excellence and success?*

I wrote these questions out because being positive about your health is worth considering. I'm not sure I've answered any of them for myself. However, it's very easy to get down when things aren't going well, and finding ways to carry on in a relatively normal manner when your body isn't working the way it usually does can be a considerable achievement of mind over matter.

God Notes
30 January 2009
Back in Dunedin

Things are struggling some days, okay on others; extremely painful sometimes, mostly just niggling. No sign of an appointment, which means there's a kind of edginess with having no "goal" in sight.- except that there *is* a "goal." Just how far away is the problem. Trying to keep my situation in perspective isn't always easy, although since I last wrote I've mostly kept on top of things—or at least not dropped into another hole.

Sometimes it's very hard going, but since we got back from holiday I'm closer to the doctor and hospital, if needed.

God Notes
31 January 2009

Dad, I seem to have an underlying irritability at the moment—not towards people, but towards things. It doesn't help that I seem to be dropping stuff all the time and picking stuff up off the floor when attached to a catheter is a pain. And I get irritated with things that don't go smoothly first time. Help me to find some peace, Dad, and to get my mouth free of words I would never have thought of using in the past. Cleanse me again, Dad.

An alternative approach to the catheter problem, from Dave (3 February 2013)

Dave

Because of prostate problems I have been wearing a catheter and bag until I get an operation. We tried before the holidays to get a valve arrangement so that I could wear shorts, go swimming and running. One nurse said it was fine, but neglected to send it out with the gear. When we followed up on that another nurse said I should not wear it. Well, we made more enquiries last week and the nurse checked with the Urology Department at the hospital. They said that it was OK for me to take off the bag and wear this valve thingy, and that apart from in bed it was OK for me to wear it all the time. I waited until Saturday to experiment with it in case it caused problems. It is *so* good to get rid of the bag, the chaffing straps around my leg, and the awareness of it being seen or being off-putting for those around me. This afternoon I have been wearing running shorts and it is so freeing. I almost feel normal again. Long may it last. It would have been great to have had it for the holidays!

The valve Dave talks about is like a tap that turns one way to stop the urine from coming out the catheter, and turns the other way to release the urine into a toilet. While it still extends out from the penis, it's certainly a good deal less obtrusive than a catheter with a tube and bag. It's roughly six inches or fifteen centimeters long when separated from the catheter tube.

It's good to see Dave feeling more positive in this last post. When I look back now, it's surprising no one ever suggested the possibility of the valve system to me, which just goes to show that people waiting for operations are often under-informed about what's available for them. In my case this meant I carried on with the bag system while waiting for the operation, and carried on having infections and other surprises.

Chapter six

Two weeks can be a very long time

Work Report
4 February 2009
And so it continues, by day and by night

It's been an interesting few days. After getting off antibiotics for almost a week, I had to go back on them last Friday. That was pretty much expected.

But on Saturday I had a bit of a surprise when I got up. You'll remember that when you're wearing a catheter, you have to attach a "night bag" to it when you go to bed. This is because the day bag isn't big enough for the expected flow during the night.

The surprise was that when I got up, instead of the night bag being fairly full as usual, it was virtually empty. Not a very good sign, but as it happened I'd only been up for a short while before things started moving in the urine department again, and went fine the rest of the morning and afternoon.

Celia and I carried on with more of the garden clean-up that we'd been doing for most of the week, and in general I was okay. Not particularly sore, and things going as usual.

However, I had a bit of a snooze mid-afternoon, and after that things weren't so good. I started having another one of those sessions where there's an urgency to go to the toilet, and the pee comes out as normal (through the penis) instead of going through the catheter. This went on; every time I got up after being seated for a while I had to race to the toilet. One time I missed getting there and partly wet my underpants.

I was getting concerned because the urgency factor was similar to when I couldn't go at all before I got the catheter in.

By the time evening came I was starting to feel lousy and the bag wasn't filling at all. Finally, I called the District Nurse department, and about nine o'clock, when I was feeling cold and not well, two District Nurses arrived. Between them they did a check to see if the catheter was blocked; it was, with some "sediment" in it. They unblocked it by using a syringe to draw the "sediment" out, and then topped up the water level to the required ten milliliters in the balloon that holds the catheter in place. I'd earlier noticed some pink flecks in the catheter tube; this was also evidence of "sediment."

The clean-out and top-up wasn't particularly drastic, and I felt much better afterwards.

However, about 1.30 am I felt the urgent need to pee again, got out of bed, dragged my day and night bags to the toilet – and wet my pajama shorts in the process. It wasn't serious, just enough to be annoying.

Got back into bed and lay there debating whether I should take a trip to A&E to get things checked out more thoroughly. Didn't. A warm bed wins over going and sitting in the A&E waiting room almost any time.

Sunday was fine—I felt better than I had for a few days. Went to lunch out at a friend's place on the Taieri where the wind blowing through the massive trees on the property was like a storm at sea.

After being okay all the way through lunch I got home and suddenly felt the urgency again—but nothing actually happened. How weird. The bag seemed to be working as normal. I'd put a pad in before I went out today, just in case, but even that was dry. I feel like an old man in a rest home.

Monday too was fine—until I got home from work and the urgency thing started again, and carried on during the evening. Again Celia and I debated about whether to go to A&E. Celia said she thought that a catheter was only supposed to stay in for a minimum of six weeks before being changed, and I was coming up seven weeks. She checked it out on the Net. Where else?

Finally at ten past ten in the evening we decided to go to A&E. Things got worse: I kept needing to go to the toilet, but couldn't do more than a tiny dribble. And nothing much was going in the bag. After an hour or more we got out of the A&E waiting room and into the ward, by which time I was very uncomfortable: painful all around my bladder area, and very sore where I was trying to pee and failing.

Eventually the doctor came, and began the delightful process of sorting me out. He decided it wasn't even worthwhile trying to see if they could unblock the catheter (the nurse had given it a brief try) and he expertly put a cannula in the back of my hand. The cannula is the tube for morphine and antibiotics and fluids to pass into the body.

The catheter was going to have to come out—and hopefully that would unblock the system.

Well, it did, of course, but to ensure things were going to continue to function okay, another one had to go in. Painful coming out, even more painful going back in again, though at least it's a brief nasty pain in each case, not a prolonged one. Still, I haven't got used to it yet, and I forget each time just how painful it's going to be.

The relief is enormous, of course. And the reason for the blockage was evident once they got the old catheter out: absolutely chocker with garbage, including the pink flecks I'd mentioned to the District Nurses on the Saturday.

After that I had to lie there for more than two hours. First the antibiotics went in through an AV line. This took half an hour and then fluid was pumped through very slowly to clear the system, which took a good deal longer. We finally left around 4.30 am, me feeling much the worse for wear, but functioning.

Celia and I slept in till nearly lunch time, having left messages at our respective workplaces to tell them we wouldn't be in until later. I felt quite good in the afternoon, and managed to work without problem.

Today, Wednesday, reaction set in, and I got up feeling very sluggish, queasy, anxious at the thought of going to work, and low in spirit. I went to work all the same, and gradually through the morning picked up some energy. It hasn't been my best day, however. Monday night's pain and anxiety had obviously taken it out on me: the body just hadn't quite got round to dealing completely with it.

Work Report
4 February 2009
Lack of exercise: *snail's pace*

I'm going to have to start taking diet pills by the time I get finished with this prostate and catheter business. I'm sure I've put weight on around the stomach; it doesn't help that I can only walk at a kind of measured pace, as though I had all the time in the world. I can't run, hop, leap, jump, skip or generally move any faster than your average racing snail.

The only exercise I've had over the last few weeks has been the work Celia and I have done in the garden; but even a lot of that was less than energetic.

Roll on the day when I'm "free" again!

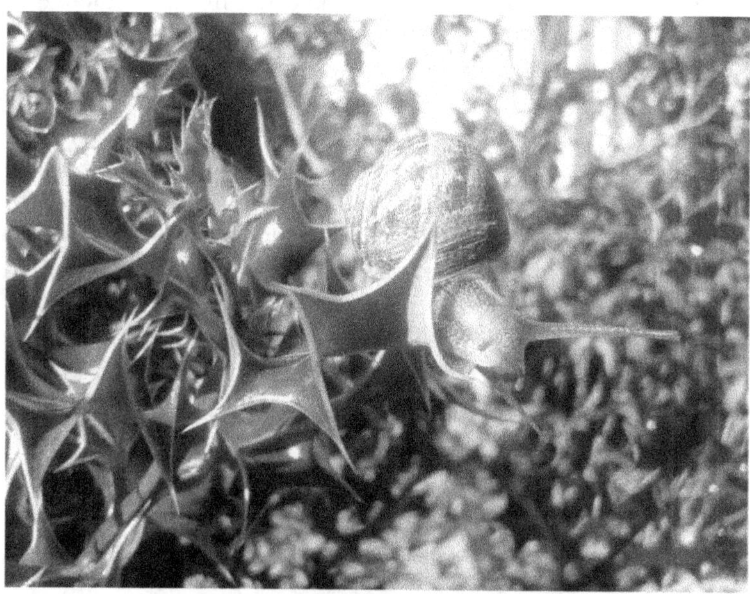

Going at a snail's pace—and adding a holly hedge into the mix.

Work Report
6 February 2009
Hacking away at the garden: let the light in

Well, after my concerns about lack of exercise yesterday, I can say that today was an improvement in this regard. During the last week of our holidays, Celia and I spent a good deal of time clearing up the garden, shifting the compost heap from one side of the house to the other, planting vegetable seedlings, and cutting back much of the overgrowth of bushes that had occurred over the last year or more. In fact, we've cut back so much of this growth that it seems as though there's far more light around the property now.

Once we were back at work, of course, the garden took second place.

Today, being yet another holiday (Waitangi Day), we got on and sorted out the front path where the rhododendrons and the Chinese bush and various other plants were all competing for space. Not anymore. Each one has been trimmed of excess baggage and there is ample room for them all to grow. Some of them look a bit bare, admittedly, but you can't have everything.

And the result of doing all this clearing and cutting and moving of shrubbery was that I got some exercise. Terrific! Maybe I won't entirely look like a plum pudding by the time I have my prostate op.

God Notes
7 February 2009

Celia's getting fed up with it all, I know. She tries to bring things into perspective, and that's fair enough and she *is* sympathetic—and she did spend six hours down at A&E the other night with me. But I know she's had enough of me getting low about it all. Dad, it just goes on and on. A friend of ours who has various disabilities tells me that pain isn't a competition, by which she means there's no point comparing my minimal pain to that of people in worse pain. Nevertheless, I still feel as though I make more fuss than is warranted. The trouble is that pain is pain, and sometimes it's very uncomfortable.

Later: Celia recommends living as though the current situation is what my life is going to be like, rather than waiting in hope for some news about the appointment each day. (I remind you, Dad, however, of your words from Proverbs 13 verse 12: *hope deferred makes the heart sick!*) Life that way would mean not just the catheter but all the gunk that goes with it—ITUs, peeing when I shouldn't, painful visits to A&E, soreness that I can't seem to do much about, and sitting uncomfortably. Good as her suggestion is, I need your help to see it that way, Dad.

Work Report
7 February 2009
Sympathy: *a friend in need*

Last night wasn't a very good night as far as sleep was concerned. I woke up at one point with the day bag hanging out of the bed because it was semi-full and hadn't automatically emptied into the night bag, as it should do. The weight of the bag was such that it was pulling on the catheter, and anything that gives the catheter a pull causes an irritation inside the male member. Celia informed me, after our visit to A&E the other night, that she noticed that the catheter actually has a kind of corrugated surface in part, presumably to ensure it stays better in place. I didn't realize this, and knowing it hasn't made me any more friendly towards it.

Anyway, I had a kind of positive aspect to the whole catheter thing today when I went to a couple's fiftieth wedding anniversary party. I met an Anglican priest there whom I know from the days when I ran the bookshop. He had prostate cancer five years ago. He looked dreadful at that time, but struggled on, even forcing himself up the stairs to our shop at one point. He expressed his complete and utter sympathy for anyone who is wearing a catheter. Complete and utter. He may make jokes about it, but his sympathy is full. Total.

Furthermore, he has to wear a condom catheter (a name both appropriate and inappropriate) in order to deal with incontinence. As one web site says, one of the ironies of prostate problems is that some men can't pee properly before a prostate op, and then can't *stop* peeing afterwards.

If it seems as if I'm making a little more of this than I might, let me assure you that anyone who gives sympathy to a catheter wearer such as myself deserves rewards in heaven. Rich rewards. In fact, one of my regular readers is also in line for such rewards as well, for her ongoing sympathy.

Comments

Bevetal: Here's hoping tonight's more relaxing and comfortable for you.

Me: Ah, keeping up with the posts as they arrive now, eh?

Bevetal: Of course....I'm scanning photos into the computer, so your posts give welcome light relief !

Me: LIGHT?? Glad they're light for someone! HA!

God Notes
9 February 2009

Thank you for a good day yesterday in terms of ease of movement.

Dad, you know the two things I'd like to see come right after the op:

Most particularly to have my bladder functioning normally again.

Not to lose sexual function.

The second one, Dad, isn't the most important—I can probably live without it if necessary, though plainly I'd prefer things to function properly. But most of all, Dad, I ask for normal bladder function. The alternatives are all pretty unpleasant or very inconvenient as far as I can see. Dad, I put it in your hands, as I have done over and over during the past weeks. Please let me know your peace in all this.

Work Report
13 February 2009
Nine-and-a-half weeks

Haven't been doing much blogging over the last week. Just haven't felt like it. It's the sort of thing that happens every so often. You just feel like you've had enough for a while.

Apart from that nothing much has been happening on the prostate front, which is a good thing, in one sense. It's been a week without too much irritation, thank goodness—and no urinary tract infections. Long may this last!

I finally gave in and rang the Urology Department yesterday, although I'd gotten to the point of thinking it wasn't worth bothering and it would be better just to carry on doing what Celia had recommended: live as though this is how things are going to be, at least for the next month or so.

That piece of advice has been worth acting upon. It takes some of the pressure off the emotional side of things at least, and you go round acting as though it was normal to get up in the morning attached to something, and dragging it around with you during the day.

I keep thinking all this must be making me more sympathetic to other people with disabilities of some sort or other; you'll note I'm including what I've got as a disability, even though, officially, it ain't. Well, although I'm noticing a lot more people who are struggling along with some sort of difficulty, I'm not sure that I'm actually feeling at one with them. Maybe I'm even more uncompassionate than I think I am—totally self-centred. This could well be. While I don't find it at all commendable, it seems to be how it is. I've worked on being more compassionate for years, but plainly I'm making very slow progress.

Anyway, to get back to what the Urology Department said, which is what I started out to tell you several paragraphs back.

I'm apparently "moving up the list." Of course, it still depends where on the list I actually am.

"We don't only do prostates, you know." Okay, so all the other urological problems are also on the list.

"The Urology Department is short of staff at the moment. One of the Urologists is sick." Yup, I already knew that—in fact, I believe he's very sick. And any hope I had that they might be sending some more of the overspill of Dunedin patients down to Invercargill was dashed. That was "a one-off." And it was for "men who'd been waiting for a long time." I already knew that too. Us newcomers shouldn't get so uppity.

"So how long is urgent?"

"Up to two or three months after you've been put on the list."
Oh, whoopee – that doesn't sound very "urgent" to me. I saw the
Urologist on the 13th January. Today is the 13th February, which
means I could easily have another month or two to go. Crikey.

I told her I've had infections galore, and antibiotics till
they're coming out my ears, and that I've had to go to A&E
again. To no avail. All that dribbled by, like water trickling down
a gutter. I imagine she's heard it from every other mother's son
at some point. And she probably goes home at night thinking it's
time she got another job that doesn't involve saying the same
thing over and over.

I have now had this catheter in for nine-and-a-half weeks.
Ten on Tuesday. Joy.

God Notes
16 February 2009

Dad, things have gone off again today—help me to get back
to some sort of coping again. It's been good to be off tablets for
a week and a half. Thank you for the relative respite.

*A bit of down-to-earth stuff from Dave on what it's like to
cope in public with a leaking catheter, dated 27 January 2013.*

Dave
Yesterday we called at my favorite hardware store to look for
a couple of items to put a finishing touch to our holiday
renovations. The car park was fairly full and the store quite busy.
I walked in and went straight to the area where the item I was
wanting would be. As I stopped briefly checking out the
displays, I felt wetness around my groin area. I looked down and
there was a large coin sized wet patch on my fawn-colored
trousers. I knew immediately that something must have come
unplugged in my plumbing system.

Holding my hand over the wet patch I went to the isle next
door and informed my wife that I had a plumbing problem. "Pop
over to the toilets to sort yourself out," she suggested. The toilets
were in the diagonally opposite corner of the store. It was quite
some distance away and I would have to work my way through

crowds of people. I pulled my hand from my groin and the wet patch was now nearly as big as my hand. "I don't think so!" I replied. She took one look, nodded, and said, "No." I was uncontrollably wetting my pants in this crowded store. I squeezed my hand against my trousers on top of the leaking tube, hopefully to stem the flow, and ran to the nearest door. (Thankfully there was a door without a checkout.) I ran across the car park, unlocked the car, unzipped my trousers and reconnected the broken connection. I sat there in the car in my wet trousers feeling as silly as can be. "Who saw me? What did it look like? Did that couple coming in the door see my wet pants?" I was aware from the cars in the car park that there were a few people I knew in the store. "Did they see me?"

I drove home feeling frustrated, sad, and depressed.

It was during the drive home that the consequences of what happened hit me. What would happen if that happened while I was standing in front of the congregation leading a church service? Imagine if I was talking to one of the managers in one of my chaplaincies? Then what about if it happened while I was leading a wedding? Or worse still, leading a funeral? By the time I got home I felt like ringing the powers that be in the church and chaplaincy and telling them that I would not be starting work. I could take sick leave until the operation, I thought. My confidence was really shattered. It was a good thing that I am still on holiday and did not have to lead a service today.

Since then I have calmed down. It has been nearly four months and I have done heaps of services, a couple of funerals, two weddings, been running, walking, tramping, working hard physically, and have been out and about doing my thing amongst people, and nothing like that has happened before. There probably are checks I could do to lessen the chances of it happening again. I will cope, but I was really struck by the way it hit my personal confidence. I know that even when things are going well, I am aware that I am "different." All the time I am conscious wondering if my "pee bag" is obvious. So it does lessen my confidence when I am out and about. This event, though, knocked it big time...for a while.

Then I heard of a colleague who has been diagnosed with prostate cancer and needs a fairly urgent operation....as far as I know I don't have that. I read on the net of a man who had been wearing this contraption for thirty years! I am not badly off really. I am just used to thinking of myself as bullet proof. Currently I am wearing this constant reminder that I am not.

It's not surprising Dave puts an exclamation mark after the words, 'thirty years!' It seems unimaginable that anyone would have to cope with this for such a long time.

For my part, however, a corner had turned. I was about to part company with my catheter.

Chapter seven

Things finally get moving—in every sense

God Notes
17 February 2009

Dad, firstly an enormous thank you that things have begun to move—pre-admission today, and op on Monday if all goes according to plan. Thank you to whoever cancelled out and gave me an opening. Dad, whoever it was, let them not suffer for their delay.

After the sense last week that things wouldn't go quickly, this is a miracle. Bless you, Dad.

Work Report
17 February 2009
Off to the op: *the goal is in sight*

Ten weeks today with a catheter, and yesterday another infection, nasty enough to just about disable me at times. Off to the doctor again, and more antibiotics. Life is so rich!

But then, a phone call at work, from the hospital. "There's been a cancellation and we'd like you to come in for a pre-admission."

Operation next Monday!

Too shocked yesterday to really take it in, but today I'm feeling better not only because of the antibiotics but because I've spent four-and-a-half hours in the hospital going through all the rigmarole involved in being pre-admitted.

Four-and-a-half hours is about three times longer than the op will take, but I felt very laid back about it all and just let the time roll by, doing Sudokus (one correctly, and one messed up), some crosswords and so on. People kept interrupting my Sudoku-solving to ask me questions or tell me things, but otherwise it was okay.

The first thing was an ECG, then an X-ray, neither of which was an issue, and neither of which took any great time. Back up to Ward 4B and my own sunny little room, with a desk that's seen better days and a bed and a couple of chairs. And some magazines. And my own private toilet.

A nurse came and did the usual things: blood pressure, temperature, pulse, etc. Nice and chatty and no problems. Everything working according to Hoyle.

The house surgeon, a young lady who seemed to be a Muslim by her dress, but who spoke everyday Kiwi English, came and asked a lot of questions about my general state of health.

A second nurse came later and went through a list of questions, many of which were the same as those asked by the house surgeon. This was no doubt to check that I hadn't been telling any lies first time around. Again nice and chatty.

Eventually the Registrar, who turned out to be Alistair, the bloke who'd done the biopsy, came and talked to me. A very pleasant and friendly fellow, even when I told him that I'd been worse since the biopsy than I was before – by a long way. I said I'd told the doctor who'd seen me a while back that I hadn't really wanted a biopsy: "Look what it left me with." I wasn't angry, just joking him along a bit, and he coped.

But he also went through the list of *awful things that can happen to people having work done on their prostates*—and informed me that they take most of the inside of the prostate away, not just a layer. Leaves just a kind of rim. Gulp.

The awful things that can happen I won't enumerate here. I'd sooner that they stayed as awful things that probably won't happen. Alistair talked in terms of "five percent this" and "very few men suffer that." Having become one of those who have had side-effects of the biopsy, I don't really want to become one of those who has side-effects from the prostatectomy.

And then they told me I might as well go and get some lunch as the anesthetist wouldn't be free for an hour or so. So I went and had lunch.

Came back and eventually the anesthetist arrived. He checked out more things and made sure my answers were still the same as they'd been with the other two questioners. Checked my heart, and said, "There's a bit of a murmur there."

I already knew this—my doctor had discovered it some time ago and felt it wasn't life-threatening, in part because many people have odd noises around their hearts. These are called "innocent heart murmurs," I later discovered. (There aren't any "guilty" heart murmurs, in case you're wondering. The opposite of innocent is "abnormal.")

Anyway Anesthetist One checked it out with Anesthetist Two—who'll actually be doing the job on Monday—and Two wasn't worried, particularly as One told Two I was able to climb flights of stairs without keeling over and that I did a lot of walking without breathlessness (normally, when I ain't carrying this piece of apparatus). So it looks like I'll be able to sleep through the procedure, which seems better to me than staying awake and knowing they're doing it.

Finally, on the way out of the hospital, with my appointment for next Monday afternoon in my hot little hand, I visited the phlebotomists' department for the drawing off of a little bit of my blood. Why I couldn't have gone and seen them in one of the many half hours when I wasn't answering questions I'm not sure.

Anyway, the woman took off a couple of vials and put a plaster over the hole. And then discovered she was supposed to have taken three samples. So I now have two patches, one on each arm.

And so to work.

God Notes
18 February 2009

Thank you that things went okay yesterday at the pre-admission, though some of the horror stories of what could possibly happen weren't exciting. Dad, I can only ask that you keep me from any of those, and that everything settles down properly after the op. I don't really want to wind up even worse off, please.

It's in your hands, and I don't expect any special favors—you've blessed me abundantly over the years as it is.

God Notes
22 February 2009

Dad, it's been a strange week—ITU again on Monday, pre-admission on Tuesday, with infection seemingly under control, infection making things very painful on Wednesday night, late for work on Thursday, a big argument between Celia and me somewhere in the midst of it all, lots of grief, and now only one more day until surgery. Dad, let everything go smoothly—you know my qualms, my struggles, my lack of bravery.

I had a strange thing happen on Thursday. It was striking enough for me to remember exactly where I was (outside the old Guthrie Bowron's shop, opposite First Church in Moray Place), and when it happened: shortly after four in the afternoon. I was just heading back to work, struggling up the slightest of hills, thinking the usual things ("I hate catheters" mostly) when I definitely heard the words in my head: "You will be well."

At the particular moment I wasn't looking for any "sign" or expecting to hear from God (as if you'd ever know when He was likely to speak), but I know that this wasn't just me reassuring myself.

So that's something I'm hanging on to. "I will be well." It's not a mantra, or a magic phrase, or anything superstitious. It was one of those moments when God seemed to speak right into my head. As He occasionally does.

Work Report
22 February 2009
Left without right: *digitally impaired*

One more sleep until the operation day, and I'm coping, but only just!

It hasn't helped this week that I've had an increasingly twitchy back, which means that if I'm not careful I can suddenly put it out, like I did this morning. Something I really don't need on top of the operation. I've got to lie flat on my back for the day after the op, so that's going to be interesting. At the moment the back's improved, so here's hoping.

Everyone seems to have a horror story about this operation, or operations in general. And those that don't have horror stories tell me all the funny things that could happen, or treat it all with great amusement—something I've no doubt done to others in the past. Justice obviously prevails.

I came across an article in the paper just now which told of a Dunedin doctor who in one week had diagnosed twenty blokes as having nodular prostates, and only later discovered that it was a nodule on his finger that was causing the trouble. Crikey.

Seemingly, the good doctor had injured his right index finger at a charity cricket match and, because he was almost totally non-ambidextrous, couldn't satisfactorily use his left index finger. He tried, however, and failed to realize he had what he calls a dermatofibroma on his left index finger. (A dermatofibroma is a harmless little growth on the skin.) Plainly the good doctor—whose name I won't mention here—has a slight memory problem as well as failing in the ambidextrous department.

Comments

Bevetal: The only operation story you need to focus on is your own. Nobody else has your story, and your story can never be a repeat of anyone else's story. Ignore the horror tales; they're no help whatsoever to you. Just remember how many people are thinking of you and supporting you.

Me: Thanks for the good advice. It's the same sort of point as the one about everybody's pain being individual. BTW, I'm wondering if that story about the doctor in Dunedin isn't a bit of a hoax. There isn't any doctor listed by the name that appears in the article. But it isn't dated April 1st either.

Yes, it was a hoax, though how it came to be thoroughly reported in the newspapers is a bit of a mystery. It verges on the possible, as many hoaxes do.

God Notes
23 February 2009

Well, Dad, today's the day—let everything go well and let your word to me be fulfilled. Thank you.

Before we carry on with my operation, here's Dave's viewpoint from the 17 March 2013, ongoing into hospital for the same operation.

Dave

In a few hours I go to the hospital to have an operation. It will be an "out of my comfort zone" experience for me. I have visited hospitals frequently over the years, but never stayed in one (apart from an overnight stay in the Emergency Department once). I have reflected on my feelings over the last months and have come to the conclusion that my main concern is the feeling of being powerless and out of control.

I have an enlarged prostate that seems to be getting bigger. If I am getting fat I can eat less and exercise more. I have some control. But I know of no exercise by which I can control my prostate. It has progressively caused me problems and brought on that "getting old" feeling. We have a stretched health system here so I have found that the visits to specialists have been rushed affairs. There's a waiting room full of people, and a waiting list, so the poor specialists treat, briefly talk and shove you out the door. I have not had a really good conversation with anyone. They just say, "We'll do (this) next" but nobody really sits down to explain.

So for the last couple of years I have been battling symptoms which were getting worse and have not felt confident about my treatment. I am an ex-plumber. I like a cause and effect world and anything mechanical I pull apart to see how it works. I don't like this gland in my body which for no particular reason keeps enlarging. I want to understand it. I want to control it!

I admit I am a bit of a control freak. I tend not to delegate because nobody can do stuff like I would want them to do. I get annoyed about things I cannot control. In the Serenity Prayer I really need "the serenity to accept the things I cannot change..." I do not like even being in a car that somebody else is driving. I used to get headaches on the shortest plane trip, I think because I felt out of control and vulnerable. If there is one weak patch in the conversations in our marriage over the years, it has been me almost yelling at my wife, "Don't tell me what to do!" There are many areas in my life where I feel I do not have control. Today I go to hospital and I will have to hand over control. I am going to be doped and have unmentionable things done to me. I will be told when to eat and what to eat. I will be told when to stand and when to sit. I will have treatment others decide for me. Because of my complaint my "going to the toilet" will be controlled and monitored. The bits of paper say I will even have somebody assisting me to shower! I will be told when I can leave the hospital. I think it is that "out of control" feeling that scares me more than anything.

I think the scary thing is I have to get used to it. That's life as you get older. Things happen to your body and you cannot change them. On Saturday, we had a coffee in a cafe attached to the local sports stadium and university gym. There are fit young people running past. I look at them and remember. I know that when I run these days after a few runs I have a sore knee. I will never run as freely as I used to run. I look on in envy. I will still try running, more slowly, less frequently and gently; it is too good to give up completely. But here is another part of life out of control.

M. Scott Peck suggested that this "letting go" process is one of the most important lessons in life. I know it is important in marriage relationships and in friendships. If you are going to sustain them in any real way you have to let people in and let go. I have learned that. We are all heading toward a final "letting go." I see older people slowly letting go their big house, their possessions, their ability to drive and their control of life itself. This "letting go" skill and the wisdom that goes along with it, is an essential part of life. I guess today I will learn more about that process. I keep trying to tell myself, "Let go and trust others." Friends tell me, "You just have to trust them, Dave. They know what they are doing." Yeah, right?

Wish me luck.

My notes written in the hospital
4 February 2009

Other events delayed me from having the operation in the morning as planned, so I didn't get into an actual bed till around one in the afternoon. Nevertheless I still went into surgery by 2.20 pm, and was out by around 4.45 pm. I think. I was pretty dozy at that point.

As a result of the recommendation of a friend earlier in the week, I discussed the pros and cons of an epidural as opposed to a general anesthetic with the anesthetist, and we decided on the former; the second was available if necessary. The epidural injections were quite unpleasant (I think because my back was still sore from earlier in the week) but the numbness was complete—I couldn't find my legs at all at one time after the surgery, and half my butt remained numb during the night.

I'm sharing the room with three other guys—one from Waikaka (near Gore) is in for a gall bladder operation. He's from a Christian farming family down there. Another guy went for his op before eight this morning and came back not long after: the doctor was sick. Operation cancelled.

Another guy had come in about three weeks ago for a heart operation. The first op wasn't entirely successful, and he had a second a week or so later. He's still unwell, with gas giving him a lot of pain. He's designated as "nil by mouth" just to add to his joys. He's from Alexandra.

After the op I felt really good; and I slept very easily. Celia and my two eldest daughters all had to wake me when they visited at various times. On top of that I got woken constantly during the night with the nurses' rounds, and other patients not being comfortable.

84

I got up in the morning and showered. Felt okay on my feet, and walked quite easily. Lots of blood in the urine still, though clearing. At this stage I still had a catheter in, though it was a new one, and did a double job of draining the urine and also any excess post-op fluid. I think.

Celia was here before eight in the morning, and then again at lunchtime. Isn't she fabulous?

My bowels seem to be sticky but otherwise okay. Had a laxative—still only just loosening.

I met a woman from Oamaru before my op yesterday. Her surgeon had flown down from Auckland especially to do her operation. Then the surgery had to be cancelled because they discovered she'd drunk milk in her early morning tea before coming to hospital. She drove back to Oamaru with her husband, and the surgeon flew back to Auckland. How frustrating.

Some geography for those who are interested: Gore is just over two hours' drive south of Dunedin. Alexandra is in Central Otago, about three hours west. Oamaru is a large town about an hour and a half's drive north of Dunedin, and Auckland is the biggest city in the country, a two to three hours flight away.

My notes written in the hospital
25 February 2009

I've been awake on and off since 3 am or so. I'm sure there was a light on outside the room that wasn't on last night, but the nurse reckoned it couldn't be turned off. My legs are aching from the horrible compression stockings, and are very hot. The rest of me is not.

Finally I got up and evacuated my bowels easily—have to use medical jargon while I'm in hospital—about 5 am. At this stage I still have a catheter in, as is normal for the first day or so after the op. Curiously enough my genital and pubic area is now very cold. Can't win on the temperature stakes. [*This odd sensation of being cold after having a pee continued for some months, and still occurs if I get up in the night to go to the toilet. I have no explanation.*]

Obviously I'm now old news: I got no attention during the night at all. You must get it all the first night, and after that you're "finished." Feeling grumpy, and want to get out of here, and back to normality.

The guy next door to me (a new patient) had a very unexpected appendectomy after being rushed up from Clinton, a town about an hour-and-a-half south-west of Dunedin. He's a truck driver and can't go back to work for two-and-a-half weeks, or else he gets no insurance if he has an accident.

The surgeons do their rounds very fast. Certainly, if they've been operating all night, as they were for the guy next to me, it's hard for them to be up and running next morning. All the same, patients need time - all of them, not just those who've only just come in.

Plainly feeling neglected. Boo hoo.

God Notes
26 February 2009

Thank you, Dad, for this operation, for being able to opt for an epidural, for everything going well, for the friendly and helpful and caring staff, for being able to pee properly. Bless you in every respect for blessing me yet again in ways I certainly don't deserve.

Work Report
26 February 2009
The other side of the hurdle

Last Monday I had the prostate operation I've been waiting for. The first op scheduled for the day took longer than expected, but I still managed to get in pretty much on time.

I opted, after discussion with the anesthetist, to have an epidural rather than a general anesthetic. Two or three people during the previous week had told me that recovery time was better and that you didn't have long-term after-effects. The anesthetist agreed, and said that he also gives you some medication to make you drowsy, so in fact you're barely aware of what's going on anyway. The epidural injection wasn't much fun, but I had a sore back already (having twisted it a couple of days before) so that may have made it less pleasant. As for being aware: well, I thought I was, but in fact I think I was in some state of being half in a dream and half in reality. I noticed the people around, but didn't notice the time going past. I was aware of people talking to me occasionally, but probably didn't respond, and apparently I coughed at one point when the surgeon was looking up my urethra through his camera (or whatever it is) and gave him a bit of a start, but I knew nothing about this. In fact, the operation was a bit of a blur, and when I was wheeled into the recovery room I wasn't really thinking about it at all.

So yes, the epidural was definitely the way to go. I'll talk more later about the following couple of days. In the meantime, suffice to say that I'm home (as of yesterday afternoon), there have been no complications (the surgeon and staff were generally well-pleased with things) and I am peeing again! And I have no catheter. *Life is good.*

I have one other memory of the op that I didn't mention here: I kept feeling what seemed to be a tube across my lap, and every so often it would jostle around on top of me. I said something to the male nurse sitting just behind me to the left, but plainly I made no sense because if he responded I didn't hear him. I suspect now it wasn't a tube at all, but the surgeon chipping away at the prostate.

Work Report
26 February 2009
Being nursed: *sleep deprived*

Hospitals are notorious for being places where you can't really rest. The daytime is full of people coming and going, which is okay if you've got the energy to cope with them, but when night-time seems to be much the same, and you don't get the sleep you need, hospital can become something of a nightmare.

The first night I spent there was okay for the most part, even though I was woken a number of times to have my blood pressure taken, as well as my pulse checked, and my temperature read. Along with this were the checks on the two IVs I had: one that went into the cannula on my right hand (the anesthetist had tried the left hand, got the cannula in, and then missed the vein—he said sometimes they move under the pressure of the needle). This cannula was doing a general flushing of the system, I think , and the other went into an extra tube in my catheter—a larger catheter than the ones I'd been used to wearing: this one had two extra tubes. This IV kept the bladder and such from any blockage. So there was water going in and water coming out on a fairly regular basis.

With all this going on sleep wasn't easy, but I was fairly relaxed, having felt so good after the operation. Plus I'd slept a bit before the night came: my visitors would suddenly be there and I'd be unaware of them. I woke up to Celia stroking my hand at one point; was awake when my oldest daughter and her tribe arrived, and then woke up suddenly later on when my second daughter turned up and was in the middle of leaving me a message to say she'd been.

The next night, however, I struggled with sleep after being woken suddenly about 2 am. For some reason there was more light in the room I shared with a couple of other guys than there had seemed to be the night before. And the nurse on duty kept coming in and shining her torch on the ceiling while she attended to the latest arrival next door to me. This meant everyone in the room had the effect of the bright light. On top of that, the patient's IV kept getting snarled up and would emit piercing beeps at frequent intervals.

I was very grumpy by the time morning arrived, and not particularly amused when the matriarch nurse arrived, woke me up, and said, "You obviously take a while to wake in the morning!"

This matriarch, however, was a wonderful nurse, very encouraging (when she got her facts about me right) and handled the whole business of removing the catheter and getting me up and peeing, with skill, tact, and compassion. And humor.

The afternoon/evening nurse was also great. She's a woman who goes to our church, as it happens, and she couldn't have looked after me more carefully on the night of my operation. She was just lovely.

My daughter and her son picked me up from hospital. I had to be taken down to the car park in a wheelchair—it's hospital policy apparently, presumably so you don't damage yourself on the way out.

Getting home from the hospital was a bit fraught. We stopped off at a chemist to get my prescription filled. Suddenly, because I was now able to pee at will, and my body hadn't got used to me being in control instead of the catheter, I had a great need to go to the toilet. I asked if the pharmacy had a toilet I could use; nope, but there was one across the road. Crossing that road (and waiting for cars to let me cross) seemed to take an eternity. I just made it in time.

Before I go on with the rest of my story, let's catch up on Dave again. Here he is, post-op, writing on the 20 March 2013.

Dave

I was so impressed with the process of the operation. I got taken into the theatre and got onto the operating table. I had the anesthetist people putting leads in me and on me and giving me a sedative. They performed the epidural which I barely felt. I turned and lay back on the bed with the operating team putting my legs and feet where they should be. I saw them lining up the monitor so the urologist could do his thing but after that I saw and felt nothing. I woke up being wheeled into the recovery room. There was no pain. There really has been no pain. I felt guilty because one man in my room had quite some pain from his operation. I felt like a fraud. The operation was a painless experience.

Secondly, I really enjoyed the company. After I came out of the recovery room I got put into a room in the ward which had three other guys in it. As I sat in my bed the guy diagonally opposite heard the nurse ask me what I preferred to be called. When she went away he, bandaged with tubes attached looked in my direction and said, "Hi Dave, I'm Merv." We then introduced ourselves around the room: Merv (early sixties, farmer/freezing works worker), John (about 80, retired farmer), and Bill (92, retired farm worker). We talked, joked, laughed, supported one another, and generally got on well. The nurses said we were the "worst" room in the ward, but by that I think they meant we were the best.

The nurses were wonderful. They all had different personalities but they treated us with respect, care and compassion. They gently asked about our needs. They joked appropriately and went about their tasks in a beautiful manner. There was one nurse aid who threw a good humored comment at me when we passed her on the way to the theatre. I, of course, responded, and every time she came into our room she kept up this good-humored banter. It turned out she lives around the corner from me and remembers my sons attending the local school. She was surprised by the number of visitors I received and said I must be a preacher paying for his church members to visit him. She never did know that I actually was a preacher, though one of my fire-fighter visitors told her I was known as "Father Ted." I was so impressed with the nurses and their care.

I appreciated the people who called to see me, rang my wife to see how I was, or texted me. It was humbling to have a wide variety of people genuinely interested, people from the Church, fire-fighters, friends in the community, and others. I felt really guilty because I had so many visitors compared with my room-mates.

The bad news is that at this stage it looks like it achieved nothing! I ended up after the operation with a line hydrating me into the back of my hand. I had a tube running into my bladder flushing out the bits they chopped up, the blood, and stuff. A catheter running out carrying all this stuff away. First, they took off the hydrating line. Then this morning they took out the catheter, and for the first time in six months I had a normal looking penis, and I could go to the toilet and pee naturally. I almost did a dance for the sense of freedom this gave me. I was hopeful of a good result, that my life could eventually get back to normal. They measured what came out and scanned to see how much was left in. We went through the process several times. The bad news was that I was still retaining too much. They decided they would need to put a catheter back in.

I asked the urology Registrar about it and he told me simply that ten percent of patients go home with a catheter and that I was one of them—I had been told the risks. He said in six weeks they would do a trial removal and see. He saw my disappointment and said, "We'll make it four weeks." I still wanted to go home without a catheter, so I asked, "What difference will four weeks make?" He replied, "Maybe your urethra will have healed by then." He then went on, ".. meanwhile the nurse will educate you on how to look after a catheter and bag." I nearly jumped down his throat: "I don't need to be educated. I have worn a catheter for six months and I was hoping this whole exercise would be an end to that." He went away to fill out the paper work.

I felt reasonably strong in the hospital. I had a catheter refitted by an embarrassed young woman med student for whom it was her first experience. I was nice to her. Then I packed my bag, walked to the car and my wife drove me home. By the time I came home I was bleeding out of my catheter, sore from the bumpy ride and feeling very weak and tired. I now know why they said it would take weeks to recover. So as I write I am feeling weak, tired, tender, and deeply disappointed. My life has been turned upside down, my usual activities curtailed and my body put through the ringer most probably for no real purpose...

As Merv said when he shook my hand as I left, "Shit happens!" But in one of my room-mates they thought they had found a tumor. He requires further scans and more surgery. Another had just had cancer cut out, had incredible pain and a long road to recovery. So my troubles are not quite so bad.

I finish with a good story. We have a lovely Indian lady at Church who works in the recovery room at the hospital. While I was waiting for the operation she took time out to check how I was going. In the recovery room she was not allowed to work on me, but she kept looking, waving and smiling. After she finished her shift on both days she called in to check on me and sometimes did things to make my stay easier. Her smile and "Hello Pastor!" brightens any day. (I have never convinced her nor her husband to call me "Dave.") But the cutest thing she did was this: I was sitting in bed on Tuesday morning and suddenly, just before 9 a.m. she appeared. "Hello, Pastor!" she said, beaming her beautiful smile. "Here! For you. I'm starting work." She was on her way to work, but she had stopped off and bought me a muffin, and a cup of coffee. Smiling, she placed these in front of me, waved, and disappeared. She is lovely. In the whole experience, though deeply disappointing, I have enjoyed the people I have met. People are good, even if "shit happens."

And with that I too leave the hospital. For me, unlike Dave, it was a permanent leaving, apart from a check-up visit a couple of months later. From then on I started to make progress, gradually recovering my old self (minus some of the prostate), and working out life on the other side of the operation.

Chapter eight

I recover, but discover that not everyone does

Work Report
28 February 2009
Walking again: *picking up the pace*

One of the things I've missed—while wearing a catheter for the last few months—is being able to walk freely, and at a decent speed. Walking has been a matter of trundling along at an old man's pace, and it's never been comfortable.

Walking comes highly recommended as part of the healing process after the prostate operation, so I'm keen to make sure I get going again. Until today, I've only walked up to the local shop and back to get a newspaper: no great task. And last night, Celia and I went for a fairly brief walk (by my standards) along the Esplanade at St Clair Beach. Though brief, it was satisfying, and I could feel long-unused muscles responding to being needed again (long-unused in the sense of nearly three months).

Today, however, we did a four kilometer (2.5 miles) walk! The WOW factor was huge for me, though not so much for Celia who's been walking to work regularly for months, and who yesterday got up to something like 15,000 steps on her pedometer.

We'd heard during the week that a walking-and-cycling track had been extended from Ravensbourne to Maia. At that point we hadn't even known there was a track at all, so this was good news. The track runs mostly parallel with the railway line going to Port Chalmers, and is between the Otago Harbour and the residential areas along the road.

Our plan, in light of my recent lack of exercise, was to do a short burst along the track and return. We didn't quite make it to Maia in the end, but we did a fair chunk of the track all the same.

Muscles that haven't been in action for weeks are now complaining, and by the time we got home (after a bit of shopping) I needed nothing but lunch and a snooze. But was it satisfying!

A bit of geography: Dunedin City sits at the head of the Otago Harbour. Port Chalmers is some 13 kilometres (around 8 miles) closer to the sea; the other places mentioned here are en route to the port.

Work Report
28 February 2009
Feeling up to it, or not

When the hospital tells you that walking is good for you after a prostate op, they don't tell you how much you should pace yourself, and that feeling good when you start out walking may not mean you'll still feel good later in the day.

After the four kilometer walk yesterday, I went home and had a snooze. When I got up I was feeling stiff in the legs—not surprising, since they've done little that can be regarded as energetic for a while—and there were aches and pains around my prostate area that I didn't like. Celia had said, around tea time last night, when I said I was feeling sore and such, "Told you so." This didn't go down terribly well.

I didn't sleep well during the night either. I've been tending to get up and go to the loo more than I would have prior to December, when all the catheter issues began, so I guess it's partly just learning to live with my normal self again. But last night was ridiculous. I kept feeling the need to go to the loo even when I probably could have managed not to. And things were sorer than they'd been for days.

One other thing the hospital doesn't explain in its After-Care booklet is how your body will feel. This is probably not surprising, because everyone will be feeling slightly different. However, this leaves you in a kind of limbo, where you don't know if what you're feeling is normal, abnormal, or off-the-wall. Nothing has been off-the-wall yet, but I haven't felt that it's all been normal either. I have to keep saying to myself: you are healing up, and healing always feels uncomfortable.

The trouble is, having been unwell for some time, you get nervous about any possibilities of going back to that unwell state again. At least I do. No doubt there are post-op blokes who feel like a box of birds and get on with life. I'm not one of them.

Work Report
3 March 2009
Recovery mode: *holding on and moving forward*

It's now nine days since my op, and I'm making progress. I'm gradually managing to get control back over going to the loo. Until now I've mostly had to make a dash for the toilet because the bladder, having warned me it wanted to go, just couldn't wait. This is partly the result of ten weeks of not having any personal control because of the catheter, but also par for the course after this kind of op, apparently.

And I hadn't been sleeping well, because, not knowing whether you're suddenly going to get a call of nature in the wee small hours, you tend to be more restless. The first few nights I seemed to be up and down to the toilet like a yo-yo. Last night was the best so far, with only one trip about 1.30 am and another fairly early one about 5 or 6. And I think I probably could have put the second trip off for longer if I'd made up my mind.

Furthermore, last night we went to the movies, and I sat through the hundred minutes or so without qualm. I even waited till I got home to go to the loo.

This probably all sounds very prosaic and uninteresting to you, but to me each of these steps are a milestone back to recovery, exit signs on the road from prostate problems to prostate normality.

I'm assuming—and definitely hoping—that everything will continue to improve. I'll walk easily, start running (as much as I was), go aquajogging, climb stairs comfortably and so on. So this aspect of the story will no doubt soon come to an end. And talking of work, that's what I now need to get on with, as I'm working from home for the most part this week.

Work Report
5 March 2009
Back to work: *cat napping*

First full day back at work since the operation. Well, by the time I'd had afternoon tea, I could hardly keep my eyes open. I should have taken advantage of the couch in one of the meeting rooms at work, and had a kip there, but I decided to go home, thinking I was washed out. In fact, by the time I'd had a ten-minute rest on my own bed, I was feeling quite reasonable again.

These sudden bouts of tiredness are fairly normal apparently, at this stage of recovery. We had a large family group around last night for a birthday party, and half way through dessert I was just wiped out. Had to go and lie down, and in fact, was so tired that I finished up going to bed at 9 pm. On top of that I was feeling unusually sore around my stomach. It might have been that I unthinkingly lifted up one of my grandchildren—not a good idea at this stage of the game. I won't do that again for a few weeks.

At least at the end of this week I can start driving. That'll be a plus, and another step on the road towards being my usual self again. I'm not so worried about getting back to digging the garden, on the other hand, and anyway, I can't do that until week six or so.

I've enjoyed being back at work, however. I've been working from home until now, and was beginning to go stir crazy, missing the company of other human beings. The kitten that my daughter got at Christmas, while it's a lot of fun, isn't all that communicative. It's begun a habit of lying as close as possible to my head whenever I take a nap. It's as though it thinks it might miss out on some important brain signals if it lies any further down. Waking up to a little cat face an inch from your nose is a bit startling. I'm not sure what it'll be like, however, if she carries on doing this as she gets older.

Work Report
12 March 2009
Update on the health: *for the record*

Things have been quiet on the blog for the last week, because I'm doing a university course (on Research Methods—it relates to the kind of work I do) and so my time has been a little more eaten up than usual.

I'm writing this post just to update things on the prostate front (not sure if that's a pun or not), and partly to keep some kind of record of where things stand at present. I'm feeling very good; not entirely hale and hearty, but getting there. I still get tired, particularly towards the end of the working day, and most days so far I haven't actually managed to make it right through the eight hours. However, I'm improving even on that score, and no doubt next week will be able to work a normal day.

Being able to walk properly is wonderful. I can't emphasize how much. The catheter was so inhibiting. I'm constantly rediscovering just how free I am without it. I haven't walked to work yet, but have twice walked halfway.

I still get various pains: the urethra itself sometimes aches a bit, especially after I've been for a pee. At least I'm assuming that's the area that's complaining. My bladder's getting used to me drinking lots of water (on top of the normal cups of tea and coffee), and I'm not suddenly dashing to the toilet, as I was the first week. There are still occasional emergencies, but so far I haven't actually wet myself.

I decided to stop drinking anything much after tea time, because I was getting up three or four times in the night. Going "dry" from about six onwards seems to be helping, apart from just making me more relaxed about everything.

There are some odd pains in the male member. I'm assuming that these are in part because of the bruising from wearing a catheter for nearly eleven weeks, as well as the natural bruising that would have gone on in the course of the operation. There's a nasty little stinging pain at the tip sometimes. A friend of mine who went through the same op three years ago tells me that because the urethra narrows as it approaches the opening, the surgeon has to cut the urethra to place the instrument inside that shaves off the prostate. Whether this is always the case or not, I don't know. Certainly it wasn't mentioned to me.

Anyway, if that's why it's stinging at times, no doubt that will heal in due course as well. Most of the time it's okay, but just suddenly there comes a kind of pinching, as though something's got caught. I just have to take care. It's still infinitely less painful than wearing a catheter.

It's now two-and-a-half weeks since the op. I'm already driving again, and in another three-and-a-half weeks should be resuming normal behavior: lifting, digging the garden (something I do all the time—yeah, right!) and cavorting with Celia. That'll be interesting.

Comments
Bevetal: Happy cavorting!

Work Report
12 March 2009
Gathering dust: *wet not, want not*

I happened to just come across an online site for incontinence products, which reminded me that one of the joys of my recent three or four months prostate-related matters was that twice we bought a pack of male incontinence pads. I was going to wear these in the daytime because, when I first got a urinary tract infection after my biopsy, there was a bit of a problem with not quite making it to the loo.

Fortunately this delightful interlude in my life didn't last long, and though I wore the pads for a few days, I soon found on one hand that the Oxybutynin tablets I was given relieved the tendency to go racing off the toilet at the drop of a hat, and, on the other, the pads were so uncomfortable to wear on top of the catheter that it was better to risk a bit of a wet than drive myself crazy with additional pain from the extra pressure the pads caused. (If you're into tongue-twisters, try saying Oxybutynin a few times in a row. Why do they give medicines such unpronounceable names?)

When I finally had the operation, incontinence pads turned up again, though wearing them in hospital in a hospital bed was a bit different from wearing them in normal life; and anyway they soaked up the excess bleeding that went on. But as soon as I got home I gave up on them. They're not comfortable, even without a catheter, and underwear does wash. So the second pack of pads are still sitting where they've been since December, and are likely to go on gathering dust! [*They were finally given away five years later, in January 2014, to an Op Shop. Let's hope someone can make use of them. An 'op shop' is what's known elsewhere as a charity shop, or a thrift store.*]

When I first wrote put this post on the blog I used an image of a product called "Tranquility [sic] All-Through-The-Night" briefs. I've since found another similar image which has this caption: "incontinence pad for men without penis holding." I'm a bit puzzled about what this means: men without penises (possible, but unlikely), or perhaps a pad that doesn't hold the penis in. In which case you'd wonder why they needed a pad. There are other photos described as "incontinence pad for men holding penis." I think perhaps someone needs to work on their English...

Work Report
26 March 2009
Groin again: *walking and leaping*

Well, there hasn't been much to report on the prostate front for the last week or so. Things are presumably improving internally, but it's a bit hard to tell from the outside. A prostate op feels like a bit of a fraud, since you don't have anything to show for it—at least not in the way of scars and such.

There was still quite a bit of pain when I went for a pee, but I presumed that was to be expected given the maltreatment the prostate and urethra had suffered, and the fact that the bladder muscles had to get themselves back together again after not being in use for eleven weeks, as it were. But at least I was peeing freely, and that was a major plus.

As well, I've been walking with great ease, better and better by the day. I've walked to work every day this week and the last, for instance. The walk takes about thirty minutes, mostly downhill, but with a short uphill climb in the middle.

However a curious thing has happened: the groin pain I had way back in November decided to return. Finally, after a couple of weeks of it getting more uncomfortable, I went to the doctor last Tuesday.

I'd avoided taking anti-inflammatories, even though I suspected the problem was muscular, because I wasn't sure how that would affect the healing process in the prostate area. I had used some Voltaren ointment on the groin, which did seem to make a difference.

However, the doctor, after pressing down on the muscle where the pain was most severe (which, of course, helped it a lot) decided that it was nothing like a hernia (as had been the incorrect diagnosis last time) and that for some reason the muscle just above my upper leg joint was under some additional pressure.

We also confirmed—as Celia has told me for years—that the left leg is slightly shorter than the other. I think this is only an occasional thing. It has something to do with my back going out of kilter at times, and usually comes back to normal by doing stretching exercises for a few days. However, it may be more permanent than I realize, in which case it's probably the reason my back goes out of kilter!

Anyway, after discussion, with me doing as much diagnosis as the doctor, I think, she decided to give me some anti-inflammatories. Forget the groin pain, by the end of the first day, the pain around the prostate was no more! Obviously the prostate and bladder and urethra all felt good about having anti-inflammatories thrust upon them. Since Tuesday, I've been virtually pain-free when going to the loo. Oh, the joy! I'm now really starting to feel human again.

I skip down the five flights of stairs at work, and sometimes climb up them too. At this rate I'll be leaping off tall buildings like Superman (though without that daft costume), and running marathons. Give or take a few months...

Comments

Bevetal: That's such good news. Must feel good to be pain-free again.

Me: Yeah, certainly a vast improvement over the last few months....there's still a bit of a niggle in the groin, but I can live with that (as long as it clears up. LOL)

Work Report
7 April, 2009
Surviving: *it gets worse*

I think, in spite of the painful time I had prior to my prostate op, that I've got off pretty lightly. Horror stories about prostate complications keep coming out of the woodwork, as it were.

On Sunday, I heard from my son's father-in-law how *his* father had not only been through the prostate op at least once—it might have been twice—but how now in his old age he was saddled with a larger catheter than usual because he'd tried to pull the smaller gauge one out (he's heading into Alzheimer's). He was literally screaming while they put this catheter in. Worse, he'd been left in the Emergency Department for quite some time with a water retention problem. As someone who now knows just how painful water retention is from more than one experience of it, I can sympathize deeply.

Another friend of mine had told me a while ago how his first prostate op didn't quite work so they had to go back in again—and then he had water retention problems as well, and couldn't get anything done about that for quite a number of hours, finally having to go to a private hospital to have it dealt with.

And then yesterday I came across a book called *How We Survived Prostate Cancer: what we did and what we should have done*. The book is by Victoria Hallerman, and it details her husband's painful journey through prostate cancer. It's enough to put anyone off having any sort of treatment—if there's an alternative.

This guy had a treatment for the prostate cancer called brachytherapy. Brachytherapy is a minimally invasive procedure that involves a localized and precise radiation therapy. In other words, there's no requirement to use devices such as the resectoscope, which are what you'd class as maximally invasive, I guess. The therapy involves the placement of tiny permanent radioactive seeds inside or next to the area of treatment.

Brachytherapy used as a treatment method for prostate cancer showed 81% to 93% disease-free survival rates.

Yes, the disease may go, but the after-effects can obviously be very unpleasant. This guy is still incontinent after six years—the incontinence is treated with medication, and of course his ability to have intercourse has been severely inhibited, which has meant huge adjustments in the couple's intimacy.

But what made me sit up and pay attention was that he had excruciating pain when going for a pee. Not just in the first weeks, but long after. So excruciating, in fact, that on one occasion when he had to go to the toilet while at a restaurant, his wife could hear him screaming from where she was seated. He finally took to biting on a cloth to reduce the agony.

The book isn't for the fainthearted, and I might say it should be required reading for any man (and his wife or partner) who's about to go through prostate cancer treatment, whether surgery or otherwise. There are obviously more options in the States, where the book comes from, than there are in New Zealand, and one of the things the author recommends is cross-examining doctors and surgeons as to why they say one approach is better than another. It may well depend on what the urologist favors, rather than what's best for the patient.

Hallerman is strong on finding out as much as possible. The problem is that many of the doctors may not have been through any of the procedures themselves, and will have a lack of understanding of the real nature of the pain that can ensure.

I'm still uncomfortable sometimes when going to the loo. I stopped taking the anti-inflammatories a few days ago, and it's been noticeable that some of the pain has returned. It's not as bad as it was, and it doesn't make me grit my teeth like it did in the early stages.

It's never been so bad that I've wanted to scream; sometimes it's left me breathless, but that level of pain has reduced considerably.

I think men facing anything to do with their prostate should talk to as many men as possible about what's likely to happen, and about what *can* happen. You find, once you start opening your mouth to other guys, that there's a lot more information out there than you thought.

Brian Turner, who wrote Please Leave the Seat Up, *documents his post-op experiences of incontinence. He'd been told to do exercises to restore his bladder muscles. He wasn't told that he could find himself barely able to move from the toilet for the first few weeks, and would have to carry a small bottle with him for months afterwards. He was never offered any sort of catheter to deal with this problem.*

Time to introduce Dave again. Here's a post from August 1st 2013.

Dave

I went along to my hospital appointment with the Urology clinic. I was hoping for some answers and some progress with my "plumbing" issues. What I heard instead was not that encouraging. It seems my bladder is damaged and I may have to have this system of self-catheterization for the rest of my life. The Doc did say that it could improve, but the tone of voice seemed to negate the positive. I can live with it—there are a heap of people living with a lot worse. He did assure me that they found no cancer when they did the operation. I have felt drained lately and had wondered if I was battling some infection in my plumbing system. They tested that and I had a phone call tonight to say I need antibiotics. The doctor did some other checks, consulted the specialist, and is sending me for an MRI scan, "just to be sure there is no cancer." I had moved past the cancer possibility and this seemed to raise it again. I am trying to forget it, and will wait with a positive mind for the scan. Life is an adventure. I learned of the death of a retired fire-fighter today. The last time he and I talked we compared notes. He had been down the prostate problem track like I am going down. He had to battle cancer. I was sad. I enjoyed his company whenever we met.

The more men I've spoken to while writing this book, the more information has come to light, and it's surprising how many men have been through some form of treatment in relation to their prostates. Men will *talk when the topic comes up; it's introducing it in the first place that can be the issue. Telling men I'm writing a book about it has helped open up conversations.*

Work Report
9 April 2009
Waterfull

A friend of mine who had the same prostate op as I did (the oddly named: TURP—the op, that is, not my friend) told me the other day that he now drinks more than he used to in the past. And so do I, but not enough apparently. I'm currently fighting off another urinary tract infection. It came out of nowhere yesterday, and, while it didn't knock me completely down, it certainly showed up those unpleasant symptoms that I remember from the December to February period. In other words, a more frequent need to urinate, queasy stomach, pain around the area where the prostate lives, and some other niggles as well. Plus a lack of energy.

Fortunately this time, I got onto it more quickly, and had the antibiotics to hand within a few hours. As a result, even though I started out today feeling under par, I managed to work through the full day, instead of having to take yet more time off. I was off yesterday afternoon as it was, when the symptoms showed their true colors.

Anyway, the odd thing about all this fluid intake is that before I had the biopsy last year, my usual day would consist of a few cups of coffee, or maybe tea, and the occasional glass of water. And I was well. Healthy.

During my catheter period I was required to drink and drink in order to keep flushing the liquid through. I suggested a more economical alternative would be just to pour several liters of water down the toilet each day. After the op I was supposed to drink great quantities of water for the same reason. My bladder isn't greatly impressed by this, since, as I said above, my normal fluid intake has been fairly mild.

Anyway, in conversation with one of the nurses from the Health Centre today, I was told that I should have been drinking a lot more in the past—water, that is, or other (non-alcoholic) fluids. Seemingly, a lack of water affects blood pressure (though

I don't suffer from high blood pressure), kidney cleansing, bladder cleaning, heart (no heart problems either), and anything else pretty much that you can think of. Which ought to mean that I should have been half-dead by November last year, not hale and hearty.

Anyway, if the only way of avoiding UTIs is to drink more, I guess I'll have to. Up to a couple of drink bottles-worth a day. At least the nurse and I agree on the sense of not drinking much late in the day—she advised drinking most of my needed fluid intake during the morning, which is pretty much what I thought I was doing, and slackening off as the day grows older. Then, at least, I shouldn't spend half the night getting up to go to the loo. The irony here is that I'm still getting up more in the night now that I've had the prostate op than I was before I had it. My bladder still hasn't got the message: it's living in the past, poor thing, at a time when it dealt with a moderate fluid intake; not this seemingly endless stream.

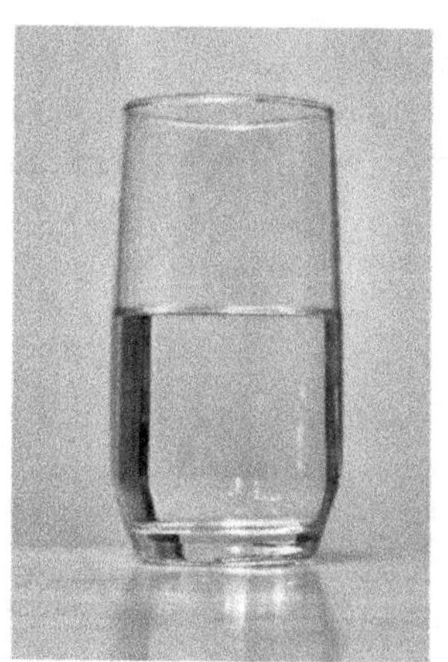

Thankfully, the business of getting up regularly in the night has eased off completely. These days I seldom get up.

The excessive drinking of water is now being questioned medically. It appears that it may have been something of a fad both within and without the medical profession for a period, and is now slowly been discarded. Interestingly, I'm now on high blood pressure tablets, but is that because I no longer take Hytrin, which you might recall one of the urologists thought I was taking because of high blood pressure, or is it because I don't drink water continually? I still walk a good deal, which ought to help keep high blood pressure at bay...

The Journal
11 April 2009

Most of what I've had to say about the prostate stuff has gone in the blog, but I haven't always discussed there the embarrassment of desperate dashes to the toilet—and not making it. For some reason, since I had the op, there are times when things just want to go, and it's a race as to whether I get there in time to get the zip undone before I start urinating—usually with a vengeance. I have no problem with the urination—in fact, I'm very happy with that—but not so much with the failure to get there in time, which isn't usually a matter of my delaying anything. It can be just a problem of suddenly discovering, after you've been sitting for some time, that everything's ready to go—merely because you stood up. As happened just now: I got up, went to the sunroom to pick up the orange peel I'd left on the table, and an empty glass, and before I knew it I was racing down the hall to get to the toilet. And didn't make it. Urine running down the inside of the trousers isn't fun, but you have to laugh—or cry. And crying doesn't seem to achieve much in the circumstances.

I didn't quite make it at work one day—though not to the extent as has just happened—and I had to somehow dry myself up before I could go back in the office. Sometimes it's happened at night if I lie in bed too long, thinking I've got plenty of time.

I guess things will improve in time, but it doesn't give you quite as much confidence as you'd like when it comes to going out somewhere! So far there haven't been any disasters in that regard, at least.

The Journal
13 April 2009

Another thing to do with the post-op stuff is something Celia first noted either before or after I'd had the op; I can't quite remember which. It was in the booklet that came from the hospital giving information about the op and likely side-effects, results, and so on. One of the points made was that men can no longer father children after a TURP. This is because the semen is projected backwards into the bladder after the op, rather than coming out as an ejaculation. Well, at my age fathering children wasn't such an issue, but I wasn't quite sure how I'd react to this pseudo-ejaculation. In the first attempts at intercourse—I say "attempts" because of the tenderness still remaining around the pubic and prostate area—there's been the sensation of ejaculation but nothing else. There's still the normal build-up of tension and that final moment of release, except that it's hard to know if anything actually gets released anymore. So it looks as though intercourse is now a kind of dry run affair—not quite as exciting, in some ways, but perhaps it has its points…

This isn't the last word on this subject. Check out the entry for 6 November 2009 for an update on the matter.

Work Report
16 April 2009
Man (this man anyway) does not live by bread alone: *going on a diet*

The eleven weeks when I had the catheter in really set me back in terms of fitness—and weight—as I'm beginning to realize. Even though I've been walking to work for more than a fortnight now, I'm still feeling quite tight around the stomach when I sit down, and am having to pull myself up straight in order not to cause pressure on the lower abdomen; or, more specifically, the area where the op took place, which still reacts to being squashed. As well it might.

I'm not quite at the stage of taking diet pills yet, but I'm certainly trying to walk more, and climb more hills and so on. Which means going back to my pre-prostate-problem days of walking part of the way home (mostly uphill), as well as doing some climbing around the hillier streets in town during the lunch hour. And perhaps cutting back a bit on some of the food intake too.

We bought a bread-making machine about a month-and-a-half ago. Well, we didn't actually buy it; Celia got it on Fly By points. But the trouble is the bread is so tasty we tend to eat far more of it than we would of shop-bought bread, which is quite bland by contrast. I think we need to avoid making bread at the weekends because it just gets swooped down on and demolished. It's not just me swooping and demolishing: other members of the household enjoy eating it as well.

So bread on the weekends needs to go. Bread made overnight, ready for a couple of sandwiches the next morning is a better option. That way you limit how much you eat. Though having the breadmaker go off in the middle of the night with a whump and a thump is a bit disconcerting.

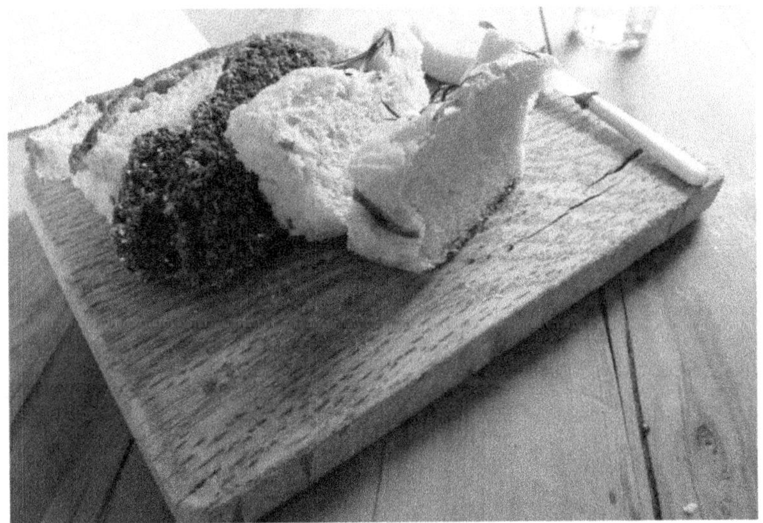

Fresh bread

Work Report
17 April 2009
Not dying at this point: *fiddle-fit*

Well, this morning we went aquajogging—me for the first time since November last year.

Nothing fell off, and there were no aches and pains that I wouldn't have had from a normal session of aquajogging in the past. So that's another step forward on the health side of things.

I'd suddenly realized during this last week that I'm no longer getting really tired at work (to the extent that on occasions I'd had to go and have a quick snooze), and when I get home from work, I don't immediately need to go and lie down because I'm so knackered. So progress on that front too!

I've got a lot more energy: I'm now back to walking part of the way home again, and I'm trying to do more physical things to get back on track. As I noted in the last entry: the weight was beginning to make its presence felt. That's something I can definitely do without.

Work Report
22 April 2009
Waiting room: *a good report*

On Tuesday I had a follow-up appointment to my prostate op at the Urology Department. Eight weeks and a day.

Because you have to do a flow-test in conjunction with the appointment, and because you don't have to do it on the same day, I opted to go in a day early. I find the hassle of waiting around for the appointment combined with trying to fill my bladder is all a bit much.

Anyway, on the Monday I did the flow-test without too much problem, and came back on Tuesday to find that the waiting room had some thirty patients in it. It looked like an airport foyer crammed with passengers waiting for delayed flights.

I was due for 2.30, but so were a bunch of others, and there was a sign saying a half hour wait was likely. And another sign saying that if you'd had to wait for more than half an hour you should tell the receptionists. Don't think there was much point.

So I borrowed a pen from my neighbor and tried—without much success—to finish a cryptic crossword that someone had started in an old copy of *North and South* magazine.

Finally my name got called, and off I went to wait in another room—one of those with a desk that the doctor discovers has none of the proper official forms, that has even older magazines than the main waiting room, and a bed that looks like someone else has just used it.

After a few minutes, the Urologist who'd done my biopsy came in, with his usual cheerful smile, and warm greeting. He's been a good person to have on the journey, I must say. Basically he just went through the notes. The flow-test (which he hadn't realized I'd done the day before, but that was fine with him) showed I was "peeing like a teenager" - a great phrase which has stuck in my head ever since.

The bits of prostate that had been removed showed no signs of cancer, confirming the biopsy results; I hadn't considered there might be any further chance of cancer, so that was a good surprise.

Otherwise he asked how the flow was going in general. "It's fine," I told him, "though occasionally still a bit painful in the muscles around the area." "And did I have any incontinence," he asked. "Nope," I replied, "but sometimes I had to go leaping to the toilet because of sudden urgency." He told me I usually wouldn't have been seen until three months after the op, when these things would normally have settled down. Through some administration muddle, I'd come in at two months.

He did an ultrasound to check the level of fluid in the bladder (minimal), and so everything was clear.

I did ask him about the rather odd side-effect of the op, what they call *retrograde ejaculation*. Apparently part of what's removed in the op is the muscular stuff in the prostate that controls the ejaculating of the semen. As a result, the semen "takes the line of least resistance," as he put it, and flows back into the bladder, to be removed with the next urination. It has a rather odd effect on intercourse, as you might expect, but doesn't stop erections, or the normal male climax, except in the case of the unlucky group of guys for whom this bit doesn't work at all after an op. In my case I missed the non-erection problem; instead I got the "problem" of water retention beforehand. There's a five percent chance of water retention, and a twenty percent chance of non-erection, if I remember rightly. Talk about playing dice.

So *home free* is the report. Things might get affected again in twenty years or so, but I guess all you can say is that's a long way off. Let's hope I either go to be with the Lord by then, or....

In general, since then, my health has been pretty good. I'm still "peeing like a teenager," and I thank the Lord every time I do. Gratitude is a thing that we don't learn easily, but a situation like this makes you eternally grateful for at least some aspects of your life.

By contrast, Dave was still dealing with his situation on a day-to-day basis. Here's a post from the 2 October 2013.
Dave

I have been waiting for an appointment with the Urology department at the hospital to learn the next plans about how they are going to respond to my MRI scan results. I was getting concerned about it because time was dragging on. Sitting in my office yesterday morning I had a phone call from the Urology Department. Somebody had cancelled out on an appointment, could I come in just after lunch. Of course I said, "Yes," and phoned my wife requesting she bring in a change of underwear—well, that's the part of the body they "explore."

I was taken very quickly and the specialist walked in the room saying, 'We don't know what is going on with you, or what to do!' Anyway we discussed the matter with questions from him to me, and mine back at him. (He is a very blunt, to-the-point character.) He told me he was pretty sure there was no cancer, which was nice to hear. He wanted to know why I still had to do this self-catheterization. He mumbled away, looking at the computer notes on me, jotting down further notes as he read. He ordered me onto the bed, "Knees to your navel, bum hanging over the side of the bed." Then he said, "Relax!" Yeah, right. After the mandatory finger test he sat down to give his decision. "Right, this is what we're going to do. We'll take you back into theatre and put you to sleep. Then we'll shove a camera down your penis (my eyes were watering at this point) and see what's going on. If there is something we can fix we'll do it then and there. We'll do another biopsy while you're snoozing too. You'll be in hospital for a few days." Upon questioning he told us it would not happen till next year—so life goes on for now. It does sound promising and he seems determined to do me some good. I am pleased that there seems to be progress.

Chapter nine

Getting to know Charlie

It was after I'd written all the stuff on the blog about my prostate experiences—expect for the very last entry at the end of this section—that I first got to know Charlie. On 22 July 2009, he wrote:

Reading your postings on bladder retention with interest—I am just starting the same journey and I am a lot better informed regarding the problem than I would have been had I not found your blog by accident. Time will tell how I go...Thanks again...Charlie

After a bit more conversation between us, he wrote on 27 September:
I have had a bad trot since I last spoke with you. Four weeks ago I was diagnosed with a nasty bug in the bloodstream which can be serious with my heart valve problem. While in hospital for the blood problem I suffered bladder retention again. I am in the middle of a tug of war between "Infectious Diseases" who are killing off the blood problem, the Urology Department, who want to give me a rebore (TURP), and the Cardiac team who want to give me a valve replacement.

I replied: This is all pretty hair-raising...makes my experiences seem lightweight! TURP is what I had. It's certainly made a huge difference, and I must say I'm now back to the kind of energy I had before all the prostate business started.

Charlie: I have been in hospital for the past three weeks while they give me massive doses of antibiotics—they have now let me come home, with nurses calling twice a day to continue to pump in the antibiotics. This will finish on Thursday, and then it is the Urology boys' turn to have a go, followed by the cardiac gurus.

Me: Crikey. It's all very serious-sounding. The heart stuff will obviously complicate whatever else is going on. We've had a guy at church who started out with a back problem, had that operated on, got renal failure, and only now, after three or four months, is he going to have a prostate op, presumably to deal with water retention. The poor bloke has had a catheter in for most of that time.

I'd be happy to pray for a good outcome on all of this, Charlie, if you'd like. Let me know if you'd like to be added to my prayer "list."

Charlie: Thanks for you kind thoughts, Mike—I will accept any offer of assistance that you care to give. Your articles and interest have already assisted immensely. Will keep you posted.

Me Appreciate that. Will certainly be praying for you.

On 6 October, I heard from him again:
My general health has improved out of sight since they defeated the "Bug" in my bloodstream. Now they are going to tackle the other problems. Firstly, I will have a Prostate "rebore" (TURP) this Friday, and then at some later date, open heart surgery to replace my damaged valve. I am looking forward to not having a catheter after another five weeks of putting up with the discomfort. I hope you are back on track with your health issues...Charlie

Me: I'm really pleased to hear that your health has improved so much. So the TURP's this Friday. I'll be thinking of you and praying for you. It'll certainly be a relief to be done with the catheter. I can relate to your pain! It takes a couple of weeks for things to settle down and get back to some sort of normality, but once it does you start to remember what it was like to be normal again.

We had a bit more conversation on 11 October:
Hi again Mike. Came home today from successful TURP rebore. The procedure was a piece of cake. Had a spinal anesthetic and was conscious while they did the "job." It is great to be home with no cables or tubes hanging out of me. I will have a nurse visit each day to give me a Clexane injection until they put me back on Warfarin tablets.

Me: I'm really pleased to hear that things went so well. Yup, the spinal anesthetic seems to be the way to go...though I can't say I was very conscious when I look back at it. I started off that way, but obviously drifted into some other state during the course of things.

That feeling of no longer having something attached to a vital part of the male system is great. I thank God for that every day...even this far down the track from my op. And once you've healed some more, you should find that peeing is better than you've remembered in a long time. It took a bit to get over the initial pain, presumably caused by internal bruising and such, but once that was out of the way, it was great.

18 November 2009
Hi Charlie,
Trust everything is still going smoothly. Certainly hope so.

I've just been talking to the guy from church who had a rebore on Thursday last week. He just came home this morning, and is sounding more cheerful than I've heard him in a long time. Catheter removed! He won't know himself, as he's had one in for I think about five months. The public hospital kept putting him off from getting anything done, so he went private (on some health insurance he had) and got the thing sorted in three weeks. That's the sort of service you need.

We caught up again two days later:
Charlie: G'day Mike..I have been home ten days now since the TURP.

Still feeling "uncomfortable," passing a fair amount of blood and some clots, but they tell me that is "par" for the course.

Being a Warfarin user for some years, because of the heart problem, they had to take me off it to do the TURP, and now they are trying to get me back onto the correct Warfarin dosage. I have injections daily of another blood-thinning agent until they get the levels right.

They tell me it takes about six weeks to get things back to normal. What was your experience of recuperation ? Did it take you that long?

Hope your friend is progressing OK...Cheers...Charlie

Me: Yes, I think the passing of certain amounts of blood did go on for a few days; though it should be settling down about now. The pain in passing urine went on for some time. I guess it was a mixture of the bruising from the catheter rubbing around inside for so long, and the bruising from the operation itself. It does subside in due course, but even now I occasionally have some initial discomfort when I'm about to pee. Nothing like it was at the beginning though.

Yes, it'll take at least six weeks before you can do any lifting, digging or anything that requires using the muscles around the loins (including intercourse). I was allowed to drive a car after two weeks, which was a plus, but otherwise I was glad I didn't do anything much during those first six weeks. I picked up one of my grandchildren one night and suffered for it the next day in terms of feeling really uncomfortable. The TURP is classed as a major operation, even though there's no sign of injury on the outside.

One thing I've noticed since the op—and this may be peculiar to me—is that when I'm lying in bed I can get quite cold around the pubic area. I don't know why that should be, because as the Registrar told me at the checkup visit, the prostate is part of the "undercarriage"—I'd thought it was somewhere around the pubic area. He meant that it was literally in the crotch area.

Anyway, whatever this feeling of coldness is, I'd be interested to know if you find that happening at any stage—purely by way of scientific research, of course! LOL

Hope you continue to recover well, and that you find everything starts to settle down. When I first came home from hospital I thought I was worse off than before. That was a temporary aspect of things, thank goodness!

And a final round of comments as far as the prostate issues were concerned, on 2 November.
Charlie: G'day Mike.... Everything seems to be much better. No more injections to keep the blood thin. Back on Warfarin again.... A little burning when going to the loo. Getting better every day and runs like turning on a tap. Going back for final check in three weeks...
I hope your mate is OK...Cheers...Charlie

Me: Glad to hear things are really functioning well. It's quite a surprise to realize how good that is after years of sluggishness. I suspect the burning will last for a bit, but it does go in time.
I saw my friend moving fairly well up some steps near the library the other day. Looked pretty energetic, and certainly seemed livelier than I'd seen him in some time.

Charlie and I have kept in contact since, but our particular correspondence about prostate matters has come to an end.

The Journal
6 November 2009

Just a comment about the 13 April entry: in spite of what the Registrar said about ejaculation—or rather the lack of it—after the TURP op, something does still happen. It's not ejaculation in the old sense (although with age that was beginning to lack force anyway) but there is still some liquid "event" of a very minor sort. The other interesting thing is that along with "peeing like a teenager" now, as Alistair put it, there seems almost a greater sensitivity in terms of erections; certainly they're more definite than they'd been for a while. Maybe they're teenage erections as well! And they are certainly working....

Remember my list of positive things for 2009? I did the university research paper as a "distance paper," meaning I didn't have to traipse down to the university for lectures, but could do it all from my computer at home. I didn't do the congregations block course because at that point I could barely sit comfortably for an hour, let alone for a week of lectures. I put on a concert of my own music later in the year, but didn't act in The Silver Chair, *only because it didn't get produced. However I did get to play a drunk reporter in* When We Are Married, *and also acted as a ghost in* The Christmas Carol.

My experience, while similar to that of many men, is certainly not everyone's experience. In a blog postdated the 28 December 2012, Dave wrote about what his situation was like before he had a prostate op.

Dave

A selfish, frustrated rant.

I had been moving furniture back into place after the Christmas dinner and found with each bit of physical exertion I had spasms of pain. Every step seemed to hurt and hot flushes came over me interspersed with feeling cold. My wife told me to go to the doctor and I grumped, "Doctor? It's because of doctors I'm in this predicament! Every time I see one I finish up worse!"

A few years ago in October/November I had a bout of glandular fever. I got over that but in the process of getting blood tests I suggested they do the test for enlarged prostate. The doctor told me the PSA reading was high and she did the usual digital test. A hospital appointment followed and after more fingers, tests, and a biopsy, they said I was clear of cancer. But the biopsy left me with some inconvenient changes in functioning.

Life went on and a couple of years later I was once again referred to the specialist who after tests asked me if I wanted another biopsy. I asked him what he recommended and he simply said, "It's up to you." I remembered how it set me back so I decided against it. A few years later, and after further blood tests I got sent back to the specialist. He decided I needed another biopsy. I eventually got this in January of 2012. My prostate was enlarged, and there was inflammation, but they could not see any cancer. They didn't treat the inflammation.

In the week or so after I discovered I was having incontinence problems at night. These were infrequent at first but by mid-year were becoming an embarrassing nightly occurrence. My GP referred me to the hospital again, and the medical staff there put me on a heavy dose of antibiotics. For a month I felt sick, but it made no real difference to my condition. I went for a consultation, and, a bit shell shocked, came out with a catheter and bag. I was retaining big amounts of fluid. The first few days were almost unbearable with spasms that doubled me over in pain. I persisted and things became comfortable.

Nearly three months down the track I went to my GP for a catheter change and he put me off till after New Year. I feel like my system is beginning to smell, in spite of all the washing I can think of. I have tried not to let the "bionic plumbing" system hinder my work or exercise, but I must admit it sorely tries my patience and persistence. I am on a waiting list for a TURP operation sometime! (They have recently given me six months' supplies of stuff so that's not very promising.) I was coping OK, but on the night of 23 December I did a lot of physical moving of furniture in preparation for the Christmas dinner. I noticed I was peeing blood and had pains "down there." We discovered on the 24th that the heavy Christmas tree had fallen over, and I tried to fix it by myself. The ghastly spasms returned and through Christmas, Boxing Day, and up till today I have had painful troubles, am struggling to sleep, and any physical exertion is causing pain or discomfort.

Out of the experience I have lost faith in doctors and the medical system. It seemed like every contact and procedure I had made the situation worse. I wonder if I would be in the same boat today if I had just ignored my problems? I suspect the medical procedures have mucked something up. At nearly every doctor's visit I have been to, I have felt I was not listened to. Whether it's my GP, or the hospital doctors, I find I have just begun to tell my story and they jump to the supposed remedy! There never has been any real discussion and questions were answered as briefly as possible. Just 'here's what we are doing... now get out the door' kind of thing. 'It's my body!' I want to scream. I wonder too if the waiting time for an op would be so long if they had to wear one of these contraptions? It is hard going when you have a busy lifestyle; it might be easier for retired blokes to handle.

I am intrigued at how many people think it is funny. "Old men's peeing problems...ha.. ha." When I asked the doctor if the catheter meant an end to my sex life, he said, "Yup!" with a grin on his face like that was funny! Imagine joking about breast cancer in the same way. All hell would break loose! I joke about it to try to make light of it for my own sanity, but that does not mean others can! It is not very funny to live through and there is a good deal of uncertainty still about the future. They always cover their butts by saying, "As far as we can tell, there is no cancer." They then say, "There is no certainty about that."

Anyway, that's my rant. I hope I improve over the next few days. It's a bugger getting old.

It's important to note what Dave says about not being listened to. I was fortunate to have medical people who were helpful all along the line, for which I thank God. However, my brother-in-law in England could barely get his GP to listen to him at all; only by persisting did he get attended to. Considering that prostate issues are high on the list of older men's concerns, you'd think that attending to this matter would a priority. He wrote: "Once it is recognized that you have an enlarged prostate and that the PSA is OK you are given pills to take, and then have to live with the effect of needing to use the loo every 20 minutes or so, and the embarrassment.'

Thankfully, Dave's situation has improved. He had another operation in late February 2014, and the Urologist "cleared obstructions and made an excellent channel." *He added, a few days later:* I am feeling washed out today, I guess I'm still recuperating from last week's surgery. The jury is still out on whether it was a success, but I think things are improving. The medical people say, "Just because you do not have a scar and outward signs of surgery do not be fooled, you have had a serious surgical procedure and need to take time to recover." I am not a patient patient.

And finally, on 18 March 2014 he writes:
[I was not] confident that my second TURP surgery three weeks ago would help in any way. But I am pleased to report that I am beginning to think that I am wrong. I concocted the following poem for my Facebook page:

I just had an enjoyable pee,
That may sound strange or weird to thee,
For two years now there's been complication
So now it's a source of great jubilation.

It is almost three weeks after my surgery and I am feeling like I am back to peeing normally, the appropriate parts of my body are functioning as per normal. I cannot tell you how grateful I am about this. I had resigned myself to the reality of having to do "different" things to function for the rest of my life. I can see every day an improvement in function and for this I am very thankful. I can look forward to normality. I share with you my joy and appreciation.

And that, for the most part, is where the story ends. As I said in the first chapter, many men come through both biopsies and prostate operations and only require time to recover. Everything else works fine. Others follow less straightforward paths similar to mine or Dave's. And, it has to be said, some men don't come out of either the biopsy or the prostate operation better than they went in. This is the reality. Yes, it's a bit of a lottery, but the odds are more in your favor than not.

Talk to your doctor, and even more importantly, talk to other men who've gone through anything to do with their prostates. Talk to men who've had prostate cancer and have recovered. I've found time and again that as soon as I mention the word 'prostate' to other men in their fifties or sixties, that the stories come pouring out. Don't try and make it on your own.

Thank you for reading my book. If you enjoyed it, would you please take a moment to leave me a review with your favorite retailer?

Or you can write to me at: mcrowl@gmail.com

If you want to read further, there's a little more to the book, kind of like the out-takes from a movie.

Chapter ten

Extras

Talking about prostate cancer

Prostate cancer, like most cancers, can grow slowly, or can spread rapidly, and affect other areas: bones, liver, lungs.

In New Zealand about 3000 new cases are found annually, and more than 600 men die from it. You can imagine the numbers worldwide.

The symptoms of prostate cancer are often the same as when the prostate is starting to increase in size, which is why it's not easy to tell without a biopsy what is actually going on. The motto amongst urologists is that it's better to be safe than sorry.

Symptoms related to prostate growth and/or prostate cancer may include:

- Peeing an increasing number of times a day
- Having trouble stopping the peeing, or getting started
- The urine flow is weak, or dribbling
- Having to get up during the night to pee, two or three times
- Finding blood in your urine
- Having pain in the lower back, hips or ribs (one that isn't caused by other back issues)

If you have a family history of prostate cancer, and are over 40, then you should be checked. If you are between 50 and 70, then at the very least you need to get PSA tests done regularly.

If you have no symptoms at all, but have any concerns, see your doctor, and don't let them put you off from asking questions.

Good news on the prostate front

Originally published on Healthmad.com 26 July 2007

Any man who's had anything to do with prostate tests will be rejoicing at the prospect of an easier diagnosis as to whether he's got cancer or not.

Prostates and Blood Tests

One of the things men of my age have to contend with is a regular blood test for their prostates. So far, though I've stayed at the top end of the range for my age, this isn't giving my doctor too much concern. And I've been on a daily tablet for a couple of years. (When I asked the doctor how long I'd have to take them, she blithely answered, 'Forever.')

Blood tests for prostate problems are endurable—most people can cope with the quick taking of blood from the arm—but they're not the most accurate of measurements. This blood test, which is called the Prostate Specific Antigen (PSA), looks for raised levels of a protein in the blood that leaks from the prostate gland. Unfortunately, while it *can* be a clear indicator of prostate cancer problems, it can also be inconclusive or misleading.

Not for nothing is it known in the medical profession as the Producer of Stress and Anxiety (PSA) test. The thought that you might have cancer when you don't isn't helpful to the stress levels of the patient; neither is the thought that you don't have cancer when you do.

Men Die of Prostate Cancer

Recently I've been reading a novel called *This Book Will Save Your Life*, by A. M. Homes, and two different characters in it remark that all men die of prostate cancer. This isn't true, of course, and in fact the percentage of men who do die of prostate cancer is not large. In the UK, for example, while 35,000 men are diagnosed with prostate cancer each year, only 10,000 die of it. That's actually a small percentage of the population.

Nevertheless, it's not an insignificant percentage. And prostate cancer is a vicious way to go. Even those who survive a prostate cancer operation are left in a less than healthy state for months on end. It seems like a small operation, but it debilitates the patient for longer than you'd expect.

The Unpleasantness of Biopsies

Equally unpleasant is the biopsy that's performed on men to check whether they have prostate cancer or not. The biopsy is necessary because of the inconclusive nature of the blood tests. It involves sticking a sharp object—like a large needle—up through the anus in order to snip, or "punch out," a piece of the prostate. If you're a bloke reading this, and you're feeling ill at the thought of it, that's not surprising. The process causes acute anxiety in many men, and may even infect them with something that has nothing to do with the prostate. Worse, though the biopsy shows in 80% of the cases that there is no cancer, it doesn't actually exclude the presence of cancer.

No wonder the prostate isn't regarded with great endearment as men get older.

Good News Is on The Horizon

A genetic test has just become available which measures the activity of a gene closely associated with prostate cancer. Doctors hope that it will make diagnosis of the disease more accurate. And here's the good part: it will reduce the need for most biopsies.

The gene test will help doctors decide whether to go through with a biopsy or not. It measures a genetic chemical called messenger RNA. This messenger transfers instructions from the PCA3 gene, and only produces elevated scores when prostate cancer is present. This makes it much more of a sharply defined diagnosis (if you'll pardon the pun).

Mostly Good News

Of course, there is some bad news as well as good. At present, a PSA test only costs around £10 in Britain. (It's free in some other countries.) The new gene test will cost in the region of £200 and isn't likely to be widely available on the British National Health System for some time. Consequently it may not be the first choice for many doctors, who will stick with the old PSA test in order to reduce costs.

Nevertheless, as it becomes more common and more widely available, this new gene test will provide a much safer approach to discerning whether a man has prostate cancer or not, and will bring much needed relief to those many men who prefer not to have a sharp instrument thrust up their rear end.

I'm one of them!

For more recent information on this topic, search for *gene test prostate cancer* on your search engine.

Some concerns about PSA testing, by Blair Donkin, health professional

I have been frustrated since 2008 by the polarising debate in the media—particularly amongst medical professionals—over PSA and its use as a test for Prostate Cancer. I feel it's got to the point of being irresponsible.

Why? Because in my opinion all it's done is serve to confuse the average bloke, who is left not knowing what to make of it all—except that medical professionals can't agree. If they can't agree on this particular issue, do they really understand it? If they do, which ones ought to be listened to? The danger of the current controversy is that it can result in blokes saying it's all too difficult. The risk with this is that prostate cancer becomes a problem ignored.

There are those in the medical profession who object strongly to what the New Zealand Ministry of Health has produced recently in regard to prostate screening information for men. Rather than criticizing existing information and requesting it be withdrawn, the best thing they could do would be to commit to producing their own plain English information. Let the critics give men the chance to read both sides of the debate so they can be better informed.

I attended a meeting of health professionals on this issue. Here are some points arising from it:

Australia and New Zealand have the highest incidence of prostate cancer (based on the number of new cases, per year).

BPH (Benign Prostatic Hypertrophy) is a disease of the stroma or connective tissue and, given current knowledge, does not progress to Prostate Cancer.

Prostate Cancer is a disease that affects the epithelial tissue, those cells that line hollow organs and glands. It occurs in the peripheral zone around the prostate. Hence the use of the digital rectal exam.

If prostate cancer is latent, in other words is not aggressive, then a wait-and-see approach can be taken.

When the cancer is metastatic, that is, when the cancer has spread beyond the prostate to other organs, then it should be treated surgically, through brachytherapy and/or androgen deprivation (reducing the hormone that produces male characteristics).

The PSA (prostate-specific antigen) test is not specific enough. Around 30% of men with increased PSA levels won't actually have Prostate Cancer.

The PSA test also produces high false negatives. This means that ten percent of men with a negative PSA result *will* have prostate cancer. A negative result does not rule out Prostate Cancer entirely. A ten percent error rate in the PSA test raises the issue of the test not being sensitive enough. Furthermore, high grade and aggressive prostate tumors don't necessarily produce PSA.

PSA levels are not independent of prostate volume (the normal growth of the prostate) and increase with age. But no upper level has been established as "normal" for particular age groups, so this also confounds the usefulness of the test.

A PSA test is considered to be very useful *after* prostate surgery to check for any recurrence of the cancer. However, while it's useful as a prognostic indicator regarding Prostate Cancer recurrence it doesn't necessarily alter the course of treatment.

Use of PSA has no impact at all on whether a man will die from Prostate Cancer or not. This is a significant criticism of the test. A worthwhile test will change outcomes—PSA testing doesn't. The trend in New Zealand is the same as in the USA where there are increased PSA screening rates, but no change in the number of deaths from Prostate Cancer.

Those with a family history of Prostate Cancer are two to three times more likely to develop Prostate Cancer, but screening these men is difficult as they are not an easy population to work with logistically.

In men over 80 years of age, *one out of two* will have evidence of Prostate Cancer, but they will die not from it. This applies to the latent form of the disease, not the aggressive form.

It's necessary to screen up to a thousand men in order to save one man's life. Statistically this is a very poor figure for any medical intervention. Ideally for a measure of effectiveness (in terms of making a difference) you want the "Numbers Needed to

Treat" (NNT) to be much lower, say one in ten or even one in five.

With Prostate Cancer the *consequences* of interventions, and potentially unnecessary treatment, are serious. Compared to other interventions, those for the prostate have much higher complication rates.

This is the other major reason the PSA screening test comes under so much criticism. If a man has a positive digital rectal examination, and then a PSA test, a test that has low rates of specificity and poor sensitivity, it's usually leads to inappropriate rates of intervention, such as a biopsy. This brings higher rates of complications such as impotence and urinary incontinence.

The issue seems to be one of benefit vs. harm.

1. The case *for* using the PSA test:
   - Can be reassuring if the test is normal, given the caveats above;
   - Has a place in early diagnosis (latent disease);
   - Is useful *after* surgery for assessing recurrence of Prostate Cancer.
2. The case against using the PSA test:
   - False negative and false positive results;
   - PSA can't differentiate between latent and aggressive disease;
   - It could lead to debilitating investigation or treatment;
   - It won't distinguish between BPH (benign tissue enlargement) and Prostate Cancer (cancerous disease). It's prostate specific but not cancer specific.

What is needed is a diagnostic tool, not a screening test.

I have discussed the above with my GP and have elected to forgo both a DRE and the PSA test.

Blair has noted that some additional approaches to confirming the presence of prostate cancer are under consideration:

*The **Prostate Cancer3** test is in use in some parts of the USA. It is a less sensitive but more specific test than PSA and has been shown to have improved negative and positive predictive values. One doctor writers: "In my practice, I conduct a second test for* *these men called PCA3, a marker that is more specific than PSA for prostate cancer and is measured in urine after a DRE. This helps to further define the risk that cancer is present and greatly reduces the number of men who are subjected to a biopsy."*

T2:E *is not in clinical use yet, as it is still a "work in progress," but it may be able to differentiate between latent and aggressive prostate disease.*

*Research is being conducted in different parts of the world, including the University of Otago in Dunedin, on **Activins A and C** and their relation to prostate cancer. To put it very simply, Activin A is believed to inhibit cancer development and progression in the prostate by counteracting the effects of Activin C which increases the development of prostate cancer cells. It's hoped that the Activins may in due course serve as diagnostic markers for prostate cancer.*

On dealing with UTIs (Urinary Tract Infections)

A couple of posts about various natural health solutions to the problems of UTIs, and my comments on them. These originally appeared on the dates shown, between other posts more focused on the prostate issues.

Work Report
11 April 2009
The U-Taken-in: *first search results*

After my discussion with the Health Centre nurse the other day, I guess I should be convinced that a lot of liquid, including cranberry juice, ought to be fixing me up well. If that's the case, then why hasn't the cranberry juice I've been drinking since before I had the operation not had much effect? How come I'm now on antibiotics for yet another urinary tract infection?

I just checked out the book I bought in Cromwell during the Christmas holidays (those joyful holidays when I was wearing the blasted catheter) and its prime remedy for UTIs is....cranberry juice, which was pretty much what I remembered from reading the book before. And, incidentally, I was first alerted to the benefits of cranberry juice not by the Health Centre or my doctor, but by a friend.

So why isn't it working well?

When I open up this blog at any of the posts, I get Google ads for a natural home remedy called the UTI Report. Of course the ad, when you get to it, is written in that long-winded stereotype fashion that says all the same things all the other ads say: we can tell you how to fix this within hours, and here are all the testimonials, and all you have to do is click here. As always they don't say on that page how much it's going to cost you (though the grocery items involved cost less than $20!) and as always they offer you a money-back guarantee if it doesn't work (it should work, right, if the testimonials are anything to go by), and, as always, just when you think you've finished reading all the way through it, you find it's starting up again, like those dreadful infomercials on TV. And if you click on the other Google ad that's at the top of the page you'll find it's basically just another version of the same thing, and eventually leads you back to the same page. Someone called Mary Jo Barton is making a lot of money out of UTIs.

You Google "UTIs and cures" on the Net, and find a page that—surprise, surprise—is written by Joe Barton, who doesn't give away the famous "secret remedy" either, even though the page looks all official and medical. Several more Google results come back either to Joe or someone else promoting the same UTI Report.

Another site at least offers some actual on-the-page assistance: nineteen special herbs and the quantities needed, all detailed out for you. And then you read an FDA warning.

Joe Barton turns up again in the next Google result. He must spend all his time repeating the same bits of info over and over on as many sites as possible. This time he gives you "Five Ways to Cure your Urinary Tract Infection at Home"—probably the same ways Mary Jo offers—for a fee.

These "cures" include firstly believing in natural remedies, because antibiotics kill off the good bacteria along with the bad. Secondly, boosting your immunity with Vitamin C. Hmmm.

Thirdly avoiding drink and foods with high acidic content: coffee, tea, chocolate, oranges, pineapple, strawberries, tomatoes, wine, soft drinks, chicken, steak, corn, eggs and sour cream. Hmmm again....

Taking Echinacea for the fourth point. And fifth, buying the famous UTI Report. Oh, dear.

Finally on Janice's Health Tips page we get some info that doesn't involve buying the Bartons' UTI Report.

Janice is into...cranberry juice. But wait, that's not all! Orange juice and lime juice. (Hey, aren't they on the Bartons' acidic list?). Raw grapes, a banana a day (hasn't worked for me, as I've eaten a banana a day for years), watermelon seeds, and finally homeopathic remedies.

At this rate I'd need to carry round my own personalized tote bags to keep all the stuff in.

Think this topic deserves a second post, in which I'll try and find some real health sites, not ones that only want to make money out of you.

Work Report
11 April 2009
More on UTI "cures": *the jury's still out*

One women's health site (men supposedly are less prone to UTIs, so I'm kind of having to put myself in women's shoes at this point, you might say) tells us the same things that the Health Centre nurse told me: plenty of fluids and cranberry juice. But they add in Vitamin C (so are oranges in or out here?)

What about the Mayo Clinic's view on keeping UTIs at bay? Well, they tell us that antibiotics are the prime approach to treating the problem, and list five common ones:

- Amoxicillin (Amoxil, Trimox)
- Nitrofurantoin (Furadantin, Macrodantin)
- Ciprofloxacin (Cipro)
- Levofloxacin (Levaquin)
- Sulfamethoxazole-trimethoprim (Bactrim)

I've had all of the first three, and have probably had the other two under a different name.

But then they go on to add: "Your doctor may also prescribe a pain medication (analgesic) that numbs your bladder and urethra to relieve burning while urinating."

Well, my doctor hasn't offered anything like that, so I've been putting up with the pain. Which, by the way, after three days of antibiotics, is still there whenever I pee.

They also note that: "One common side effect of urinary tract analgesics is discolored urine—bright blue or orange." That's interesting: I seem to remember I managed to have purple urine *without* having any analgesic. I wrote about this on 29 December.

The Mayo people have another page in which they discuss lifestyle and home remedies. "Avoid coffee, alcohol, and soft drinks containing citrus juices and caffeine until your infection has cleared," they say. Hmmm. And, of course, drink the ubiquitous cranberry juice!

There are only a few other results from Google on the subject of UTI health and none of them vary much from what I've already written. Basically, you can go via some herbal treatment or via antibiotics (and cranberry juice). There's little else to do— unless you want to pay for the famous UTI Report.

One last note: tests to show cranberry juice is actually effective in treating UTIs haven't been conclusive. It obviously does no harm; neither is it guaranteed to do any good. In other words, the jury is still out on cranberry juice and UTIs, even though it seems everyone is recommending it!

Comment

Anonymous: Yes, I am suspicious that you MUST pay for this UTI report to find out the "secret" cure. Both of my parents are medical workers, and they can't recommend anything more than the usual antibiotics and cranberry juice. However, as you say, I had another doctor tell me that cranberry juice is fairly acidic and therefore may not be all that helpful.

Just to pass on some useful info, below I've listed a few other (mostly anecdotal) remedies that friends and my parents' patients have found helpful, some of which may seem a bit weird—

- Cranberry capsules
- Zinc and Garlic supplement capsules

- Dissolving bicarbonate of soda in your drink at regular intervals
- Having a hot bath and not holding back if you want to pee in there (mmm, nice)
- Keeping your crotch warm, by using a hand warmer or wearing multiple pairs of underwear.
- Hope this helps!

Me: Interesting bunch of "remedies." Can't say I've tried the zinc and garlic, or the bicarb, but the others have all been tested and tried! LOL

Anyway, since I wrote this a few weeks ago things have improved greatly, and I certainly haven't had any further UTIs. I have been using the fizzy cranberry capsules in water—pretty bland, I must say. And I keep on drinking far more than I used to, so I guess it's all good!

Thanks for your comments.

Acknowledgements

I want to acknowledge the help of my longstanding friend Richard who had a similar experience to mine, and was able to encourage me a good deal when I was going through the things I've written about in this book. And Arnold, who first alerted me to the awfulness of water retention.

I've also learned more about the experience of dealing with prostate issues from my brother-in-law, from cousins, and from friends who've come through the process alive but not necessarily intact.

Thanks also to two particular people who commented on my blog and gave permission for their comments to be included in this book: Bevetal and Katyzzz. Another comment was made by someone who wished to remain anonymous.

Considerable thanks are due to Jason Goroncy, who edited this book in exceptional detail. If there are still any issues with it it's because I didn't always follow his sound advice.

And last, but by no means least, thanks to my precious wife, Celia, who endured my moans and groans, and was always there when I needed her.

Portions of this book first appeared as blog posts on the now defunct blog, *Work Report*, in 2008 and 2009. They have been edited and revised. *Work Report.net* was a blog run under the umbrella of *Orble.com*, a "community of bloggers who provide an independent source of news, features, opinion, and entertainment."

A few posts relating to the holiday period in early 2009 were originally published on Mike Crowl's Travel Diary. These also have been revised and edited.

Dave's blog posts were originally published on his blog, *JC's Helper*, and are used with his permission. The versions in this book have been abridged from the originals.

Please Leave the Seat Up!: confronting my prostate cancer with humor by Brian Turner is available via Amazon.co.uk. When I first came across this book, I didn't get round to reading it. It might have been helpful if I'd done so. Nevertheless, I've now read it, and recommend it highly to anyone facing *anything* to do with the prostate, not just prostate cancer.

The book, *Natural Remedies that Really Work,* by Dr Shaun Holt and Iona MacDonald, is published by Craig Potton Publishing, Nelson, New Zealand.

How We Survived Prostate Cancer: what we did and what we should have done, by Victoria Hallerman, is available via Amazon.com.

Photo and drawing credits

Digital rectal examination *drawing by Alan Hoofring. Drawing now in public domain, courtesy of Wikimedia Commons.*

Casting Call *photo used with the permission of Ryan Ozawa.*

Quails *photo by 'Steinerdoom.' Photo now in public domain, courtesy of Wikimedia Commons.*

Please Leave the Seat Up*, cover used with the permission of the author's wife, Carol Turner.*

Benign prostatic hyperplasia *by an unknown illustrator, courtesy Wikimedia Commons.*

Insertion of the catheter *by Pöllö, courtesy of Wikimedia Commons.*

Disability Toilet *by Jean Louis Zimmerman, courtesy of Wikimedia Commons.*

Transurethral Resector*, photo by Ramonduran, courtesy of Wikimedia Commons.*

Natural Remedies That Really Work*, cover used with the permission of Craig Potton Publishing.*

Snail on holly hedge*, photo taken by Mike Crowl.*

Glass half full*, by Derek Jansen. Photo now in public domain, courtesy of Wikimedia Commons.*

Fresh bread*, by Ewan Munro, courtesy of Wikimedia Commons.*

The photo of Mike Crowl was taken by Steve Murphy.

About the Author

Mike Crowl has published articles, a weekly newspaper column, blog posts, and short stories. He is also as a composer of songs and piano pieces, and has taken part in several theatrical productions in the 21st century.

He has been happily married for nearly forty-five years, has five grown-up children and twelve (going on thirteen) grandchildren. Though born in Melbourne, Australia, he has lived most of his life in Dunedin, New Zealand.

This is his second book. Mike has also written three fantasies for children aged 7-12 (roughly) in a series called *Grimhilderness*. These can also be read as standalone titles.

Grimhilda! a fantasy for children and their parents (2014)

The Mumbersons and the Blood Secret (2014)

The Disenchanted Wizard (2017)

A fourth book in the *Grimhilderness* series is in the pipeline.

These children's fantasies are currently available as Kindle e-books via Amazon.com

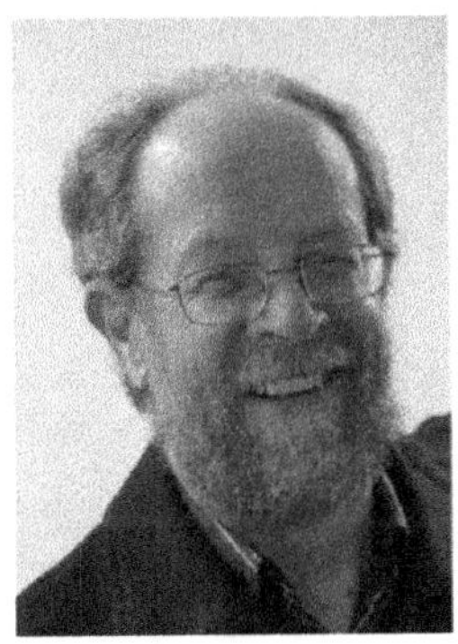